A Beginner's Guide to Medical Application Development with Deep Convolutional Neural Networks

This book serves as a source of introductory material and reference for medical application development and related technologies by providing the detailed implementation of cutting-edge deep learning methodologies. It targets cloud-based advanced medical application developments using open-source Python-based deep learning libraries. It includes code snippets and sophisticated convolutional neural networks to tackle real-world problems in medical image analysis and beyond.

Features:

- Provides programming guidance for creation of sophisticated and reliable neural networks for image processing.
- Incorporates the comparative study on GAN, stable diffusion, and its application on medical image data augmentation.
- Focuses on solving real-world medical imaging problems.
- Discusses advanced concepts of deep learning along with the latest technology such as GPT, stable diffusion, and ViT.
- Develops applicable knowledge of deep learning using Python programming, followed by code snippets and OOP concepts.

This book is aimed at graduate students and researchers in medical data analytics, medical image analysis, signal processing, and deep learning.

A Beginner's Guide to Medical Application Development with Deep Convolutional Neural Networks

Snehan Biswas, Amartya Mukherjee, and
Nilanjan Dey

CRC Press
Taylor & Francis Group
Boca Raton London New York

CRC Press is an imprint of the
Taylor & Francis Group, an **informa** business

Designed cover image: Shutterstock

First edition published 2025
by CRC Press
2385 NW Executive Center Drive, Suite 320, Boca Raton FL 33431

and by CRC Press
4 Park Square, Milton Park, Abingdon, Oxon, OX14 4RN

CRC Press is an imprint of Taylor & Francis Group, LLC

ISBN: 9781032589275 (hbk)
ISBN: 9781032598291 (pbk)
ISBN: 9781003456476 (ebk)

DOI: 10.1201/9781003456476

Typeset in Times
by Newgen Publishing UK

Contents

Preface

The field of medicine generates vast amounts of data every day, ranging from patient records to medical imaging scans. This data has the potential to revolutionize the way we diagnose and treat diseases, but extracting meaningful insights from it can be a daunting task. Traditional methods of data analysis are often limited by their inability to process complex and heterogeneous data, leading to missed opportunities for critical diagnoses and treatment decisions.

In recent years, deep neural networks (DNNs) have emerged as a powerful tool for analyzing medical data. These networks are capable of learning complex patterns in data, and can be trained to identify subtle features that traditional methods may miss. With the ability to process large amounts of data quickly and accurately, DNNs offer a promising avenue for improving medical diagnosis and treatment.

This book aims to provide a comprehensive introduction to the use of DNNs for medical data analysis. The book is intended for a wide audience, including healthcare professionals, data scientists, researchers, and students. It covers the basics of neural networks and deep learning, and provides a detailed overview of the various types of networks that can be used for medical data analysis. The book also includes case studies and practical examples of how DNNs have been used to diagnose and treat a range of medical conditions.

Chapter 1 provides an overview of the basics of neural networks and deep learning. It covers the fundamentals of how neural networks work and how they can be used to learn from data. The chapter also explores different types of deep learning architectures and how they can be used for medical data analysis.

Chapter 2 focuses on the details about a special type of neural network, known as the convolutional neural network (CNN), and how it can solve the problems of image analysis by learning different features of the training images. The chapter also provides an idea about some of the recent state-of-the-art models that have been developed by researchers all around the world.

Chapter 3 explores how a sophisticated CNN can be designed using Python for solving the recognition of pneumonia category using chest X-ray images dataset. The chapter deals with details about the dataset preparation along with the designing of the CNN using Tensorflow library and OpenCV-Python.

Chapter 4 focuses on the use of DNNs for personalized medical imagery data analysis on a small scale. The main objective of this chapter is to guide the readers in solving small-scale image recognition problems using customized feature extractor along with traditional machine learning algorithms. We have demonstrated the usage of a state-of-the-art model known as the VGG model as the feature extractor along with a random forest classifier.

Chapter 5 covers the ethical considerations involved in designing an ensemble system of CNNs that will solve the task of recognizing malarial cell images. The chapter presents in detail about the dataset creation and the techniques of image data tensor formation; the CNNs have been designed using Tensorflow and Keras from scratch.

Chapter 6 guides the readers in understanding the complicated concept of deep learning by using a very easy approach. The chapter deals with what a CNN learns during its training and also the designed system is incorporated with an auto-encoder. This chapter presents the problem of performing medical image data reconstruction and hence during this process the learned features of the CNN are visualized. The chapter helps the readers in creating the code for the system from scratch.

Chapter 7 tackles an advanced problem in deep learning, the concept of image super resolution in medical domain. The chapter helps the readers in understating a sophisticated neural network system known as Super Resolution Generative Adversarial Neural Network (SR-GANN), via simple code snippets written in Python. The system data creation for training is also designed using Python from scratch.

In conclusion, this book provides a comprehensive introduction to the use of CNNs for medical data analysis. It covers the basics of neural networks and deep learning, and provides a detailed overview of the different types of networks that can be used for medical data analysis. The book includes case studies and practical examples of how CNNs have been used to diagnose and treat a range of medical conditions.

The book highlights the potential of using DNNs for medical data analysis and how it can revolutionize the way we diagnose and treat diseases.

Chapters in the book cover topics such as CNNs for image analysis, personalized medical imagery data analysis, ethical considerations, and advanced problems in deep learning.

Acknowledgments

The creation of this book would not have been possible without the unwavering guidance and support of my beloved parents, Mr. Santanu Biswas and Mrs. Sudeshna Biswas. I am also grateful to my maternal grandmother, who not only taught me the fundamentals of education during my childhood but also supported me throughout my entire academic journey. I extend my gratitude to all of my teachers who not only assisted me but also provided guidance during the challenging periods and fluctuations in my life. Creating a visually sophisticated and eye-catching book was a challenging task that required significant effort. I am deeply grateful to my teammate, Miss Sudipa Dutta, who not only contributed wonderful and captivating illustrations for this book but also provided constant support throughout its completion. These illustrations are sure to delight and engage readers, and I owe it all to Miss Dutta's skill and dedication.

Snehan Biswas

I would like to thank my wife Eshita and my only son Eehaan. Without your support this book is not possible.

Amartya Mukherjee

I would like to thank my wife and my little princess. Without your mental support this book might not be possible.

Nilanjan Dey

About the Authors

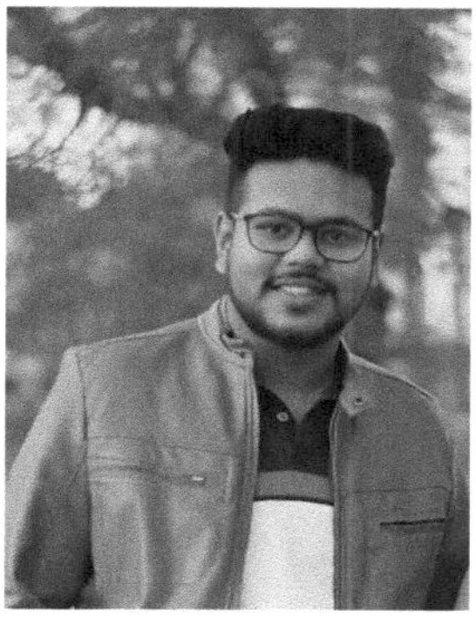

Snehan Biswas is Senior System Analyst in the Department of Machine Learning and IoT, IEMA Research & Development Private Limited, India. He is a graduate in Electronics and Communication Engineering from the University of Engineering and Management, Kolkata, India. His research interest includes Medical Image Processing, Machine Learning, Deep Learning, DevOps, and Edge and Cloud Computing. He has written several research articles in the field of deep learning, machine learning, and cloud computing.

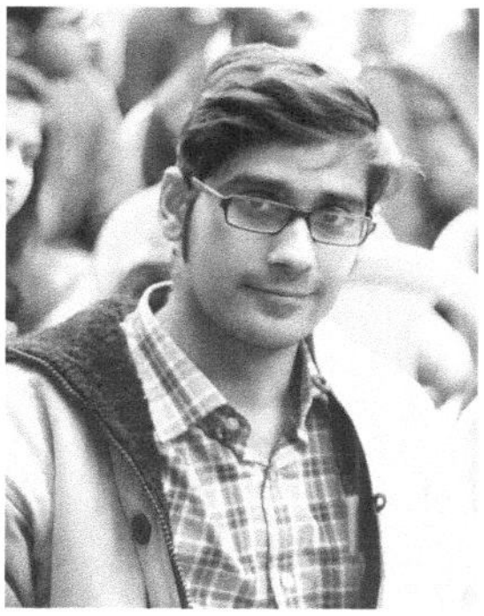

Amartya Mukherjee is Head of the Department in the Department of CSE (AIML), Institute of Engineering & Management, Kolkata, India. He is currently doing his research at the Maulana Abul Kalam Azad University of Technology, West Bengal, India. He holds a master's degree in Computer Science and Engineering from the NIT, Durgapur, West Bengal, India. His research interest includes machine learning, deep learning, IoT, wireless communication, sensor networks, and healthcare. He has written many research articles and books in the domain of IoT, machine learning, biomedical systems, and sensor networks.

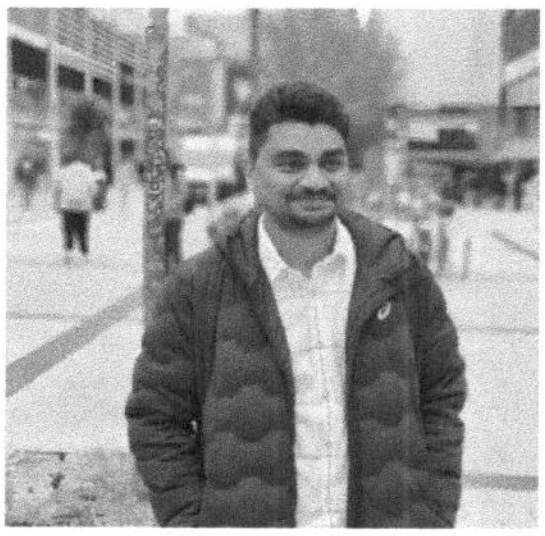

Nilanjan Dey is Associate Professor in the Department of Computer Science and Engineering at Techno International New Town, New Town, Kolkata, India. He is a visiting fellow of the University of Reading, UK. He is a visiting professor at Wenzhou Medical University, China and Duy Tan University, Vietnam. He was an honorary visiting scientist at Global Biomedical Technologies Inc., CA, USA (2012–2015). He was awarded his PhD from Jadavpur University in 2015. He has authored/edited more than 45 books with several reputed publishers, and published more than 300 papers. His main research interests include medical imaging, machine learning, computer-aided diagnosis, and data mining. He is the Indian Ambassador of International Federation for Information Processing (IFIP) – Young ICT Group. Recently, he has been awarded as one among the top ten most published academics in the field of computer science in India (2015–2017).

1 Introduction to Medical Data and Image Analysis

1.1 INTRODUCTION

In the realm of medical disease diagnosis, medical imaging has become an indispensable tool. Recent advancements in artificial intelligence, machine learning, and deep learning algorithms present a remarkable opportunity for healthcare professionals and researchers to achieve early detection of diseases, such as pneumonia, cancer, and so on. Medical imaging has a long history, with X-ray imaging being the prevalent method in earlier times for diagnosing orthopedic disorders and tumors. Researchers engage in various levels of analysis of diverse medical image datasets, and the insights derived from this analysis aid in accurate medical diagnoses. In the medical domain, data can assume various forms, including pathological data such as blood glucose levels, hormonal ranges, blood cell counts, vitamin and mineral levels in the blood, C-reactive protein levels, and various factor parameters. In addition, medical data can also be acquired from sensing devices like electrocardiogram (ECG), pulse rate, oxygen saturation level, electroencephalogram data, and blood pressure, often through noninvasive methods. An intriguing innovation in sensing technology is sensor pills—tiny robotic pills that can be ingested by humans. In some cases, these pills are used for endoscopy imaging. Notably, the field of medical image analysis has witnessed significant progress. Systems that autonomously learn features from data have gradually supplanted systems reliant on manually crafted features. Prior to the breakthrough brought about by AlexNet, various methods for feature learning were commonly employed, as thoroughly explored by various other computer scientists and researchers. These methods encompassed a wide range, from dictionary techniques and principal component analysis to picture patch clustering, among others.

Tuberculosis (TB) s is a particularly dire disease with a high mortality rate, primarily affecting the lungs due to *Mycobacterium tuberculosis* infection. The conventional approach to diagnosing TB involves a battery of tests, including blood tests, chest X-rays (CXR), sputum smear microscopy, culture tests, skin tests, and more. Misclassification of CXR images of TB as other diseases with similar radiological characteristics can lead to incorrect diagnosis and treatment. In the era of artificial intelligence, machine learning (ML), and deep learning (DL), these techniques have enabled early and accurate detection of TB.

DOI: 10.1201/9781003456476-1

1.2 THE CLASSICAL VS MODERN MEDICAL IMAGING TECHNOLOGY

1.2.1 The History of ECG

In May 1887, a groundbreaking moment occurred at St. Mary's Hospital in London when Augustus Waller utilized a mercury capillary electrometer to record the first ECG from an intact human heart. The initial tracing yielded only two distorted deflections, which were considered unsatisfactory. Willem Einthoven (1860–1927), a physiology professor at the University of Leiden in the Netherlands, embarked on his own journey of ECG research using a similar mercury capillary electrometer.

Through mathematical refinements, Einthoven successfully corrected the distortions inherent to the device. By the end of the century, he was able to produce precise representations of ECGs. Einthoven went on to introduce his own design of a string galvanometer, significantly enhancing the quality of ECG recordings. His initial paper on the string galvanometer was published in 1901, followed by a more comprehensive description in 1903, which included reports of ECGs recorded with the new instrument. Remarkably, it wasn't until 2002, the centennial of this discovery, that Willem Einthoven's string galvanometer was used to clinically record ECGs in a practical manner.

In a 1906 article on the "télécardiogram," Einthoven's stationary equipment required the telephonic transmission of ECG data from the physiology laboratory to the Academic Hospital's clinic, which was approximately a mile away. This report featured numerous ECG patterns and arrhythmias. Einthoven also introduced the triaxial bipolar system, which incorporated three limb leads, and established an electrocardiographic standardization system that continues to be in use today.

Traditionally, the term "ECG" referred to a 12-lead ECG recorded with the patient lying down, as described below. While some smartwatches can also record ECGs, other devices like Holter monitors are capable of capturing the heart's electrical activity. ECG signals can be obtained using various tools in diverse clinical scenarios.

1.2.2 The History of X-Ray

On November 8, 1895, during his experiments involving Lenard tubes and Crookes tubes, Wilhelm Röntgen, a German physics professor, made a serendipitous discovery—X-rays. Fascinated by this newfound phenomenon, he embarked on an extensive investigation into its characteristics.

Wilhelm Röntgen was awarded the inaugural Nobel Prize in Physics, nevertheless, due to Röntgen's decision to destroy his laboratory notes upon his passing, various accounts of his discovery have surfaced. Nonetheless, one plausible reconstruction by his biographers is as follows: While investigating cathode rays emitted from a Crookes tube covered with light-blocking black cardboard, Röntgen noticed a faint green glow approximately one meter away on a fluorescent screen coated with barium platinocyanide.

He surmised that this glow was caused by imperceptible rays emanating from the tube. Remarkably, these rays possessed the ability to penetrate through books and documents on his desk. Röntgen became deeply engrossed in a systematic study of these enigmatic rays and published his findings just two months after their initial detection. Furthermore, some publications linked this novel form of radiation to occult and supernatural concepts, such as telepathy, contributing to the sensationalism surrounding this groundbreaking discovery.

1.2.3 Magnetic Resonance Imaging (MRI) and Computed Tomography (CT) Scan

MRI employs a powerful magnetic field, radio waves, and computer technology to generate highly accurate images of the body's internal structures [1, 2]. This advanced technique finds applications in various medical scenarios within the chest, abdomen, and pelvis, aiding in both diagnosis and the assessment of treatment effectiveness. In cases of pregnancy, doctors may employ body MRI to closely monitor the health of the unborn child, offering a noninvasive approach. Medical practitioners rely on MRI as a safe and noninvasive means to detect medical conditions. This imaging process does not involve radiation, such as X-rays. Instead, it utilizes a strong magnetic field, radiofrequency pulses, and sophisticated computer algorithms to produce detailed images of the body's internal anatomy. These precise MRI images enable healthcare professionals to identify and assess various diseases and conditions with a high degree of accuracy (Figure 1.1).

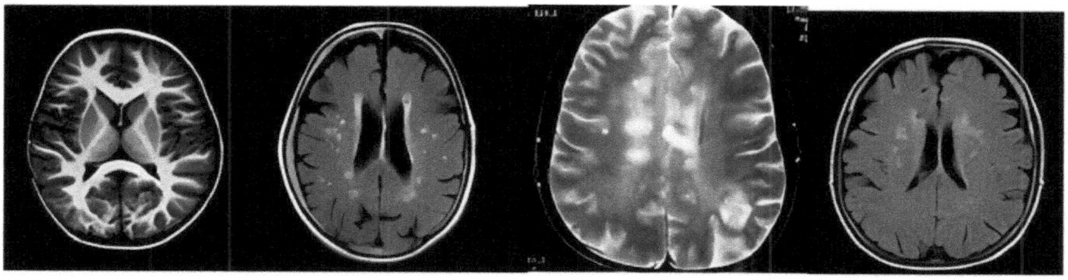

FIGURE 1.1 MRI image snapshot of the brain. (Source: Kaggle.com).

Body MRI is a diagnostic technique used to assess the condition of organs within the chest and abdomen, including the adrenal glands, kidneys, spleen, liver, biliary tract, and intestines. Reproductive organs like the uterus and ovaries in females and the prostate gland in males, along with the bladder, collectively constitute the pelvic organs. Additionally, it can be used to examine body fluids, including MR angiography, and lymph glands. Doctors employ MRI scans to aid in the diagnosis and monitoring of various illnesses such as malignancies in the chest, abdomen, or pelvis, as well as disorders affecting the pancreas, bile ducts, liver diseases, including cirrhosis, and inflammatory bowel diseases such as Crohn's disease and ulcerative colitis, among other heart conditions, including congenital heart disease.

Before undergoing an MRI, it's necessary to change into a hospital gown to adhere to safety regulations pertaining to the strong magnetic field and to prevent artifacts from appearing in the final images. Dietary and medication restrictions before an MRI may vary depending on the specific test and facility. Generally, unless otherwise instructed by your doctor, you can continue with your regular eating and medication regimen. In some MRI examinations, a contrast substance is injected. If you have allergies or asthma related to substances, medications, foods, or the environment, your doctor may inquire about them. One common contrast agent used in MRI is gadolinium, which is utilized when patients are allergic to iodine contrast.

For female patients, it's important to disclose pregnancy to the doctor and the technician. MRI scans have been used since the 1980s, and there have been no reports of adverse effects on expectant mothers or their unborn children due to MRI exposure. However, it's worth noting that the infant will be exposed to a strong magnetic field, so MRI during the first trimester is generally avoided unless the potential benefits outweigh any potential risks. Gadolinium contrast should only be administered to pregnant women when absolutely necessary. It's important to note that MRI scans do not involve radiation, unlike X-rays and CT scans. Instead, MRI realigns hydrogen atoms already present in the body using radio waves, causing no chemical alterations to tissues. These realigned hydrogen atoms emit varying amounts of energy depending on their tissue context, which is captured by the scanner and used to create images. CT scans offer superior detail compared to conventional X-rays. In a regular X-ray, a beam of radiation is directed at the specific part of the body under examination. After passing through the skin, bone, muscle, and other tissues, the X-ray beam is captured by a plate positioned behind the body part. While a standard X-ray can provide valuable information, it lacks the ability to reveal internal organs and structures in great detail. During a CT scan, the X-ray source revolves around the body in a circular motion, providing a wealth of data and allowing for multiple views of the same organ or structure. This X-ray data is transmitted to a computer, which processes and displays it on a monitor in two dimensions. Recent advancements in technology and computer software even enable the creation of three-dimensional graphics. CT scans find applications in diagnosing cancers, investigating internal bleeding, examining other internal injuries or damage, and facilitating tissue or fluid biopsies (Figure 1.2).

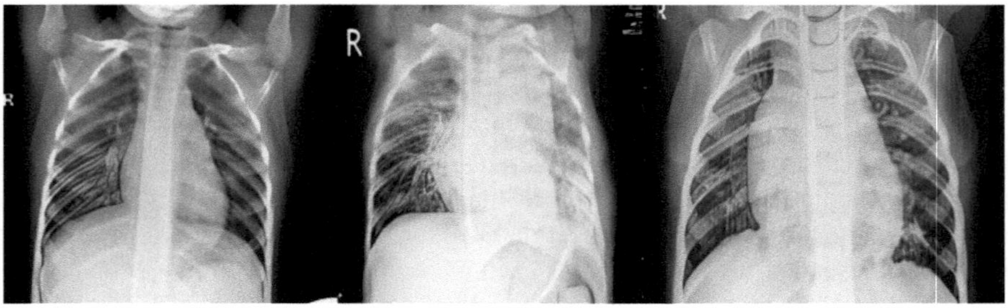

FIGURE 1.2 CT scan image snapshot of the lungs to detect COVID-19 and pneumonia. (Source: Kaggle.com).

Prior to the procedure, your doctor will let you know about this. You must inform your doctor if you have ever experienced a reaction to any contrast material or if you have any renal issues. Iodinated contrast is not regarded as being contraindicated in the presence of a known seafood allergy. Tell your doctor if you have any illnesses or disorders that have recently plagued you.

Positron emission tomography (PET) is an imaging procedure designed to provide insights into the metabolic or biochemical functioning of your tissues and organs. During a PET scan, a radioactive substance, known as a tracer, is used to highlight both normal and abnormal metabolic activities. In many cases, a PET scan can detect irregular tracer metabolism in conditions even before they become apparent on other imaging tests like CT scans or MRI. This capability to identify early metabolic changes sets PET scans apart in the realm of medical diagnostics.

1.3 MEDICAL IMAGE PREPROCESSING

Prior to utilizing medical data, it is essential to perform preprocessing to ensure its suitability [3, 4]. Medical data can sometimes contain noise and may not be suitable for artificial intelligence (AI)-based analysis. Therefore, efficient data preprocessing is necessary to prepare the data for use with AI tools. It involves capturing X-ray images from multiple angles and merging them to create detailed images that offer more comprehensive information than standard X-ray images. This method allows for the detection of abnormalities in a patient's tissues, veins, or bones. Consequently, it enhances the accuracy of diagnosis and guides appropriate treatment. To delve into preprocessing, it's crucial to understand certain well-known file formats. Let's begin by discussing the DICOM format, which stands for Digital Imaging and Communication in Medicine. Files in this format are commonly saved with the ".dcm" file extension. DICOM serves as both a communication protocol and a file format, enabling the storage of both patient-specific information and medical data, such as MRI and ultrasound images, within a single file. Unlike formats like Portable Network Graphics (PNG) file or Joint Photographic Experts Group (JPEG) file, DICOM provides comprehensive patient data, including windowing intervals for the image and additional metadata.

In essence, DICOM format encapsulates more detailed patient information and keeps all the data in one place. It facilitates the exchange of information between devices that support DICOM, streamlining the sharing and management of medical data. During the preparation phases of image data, five steps are required, which are as follows: converting to Hounsfield unit (HU), eliminating noise, correcting for tilt, cropping images, and padding. These preprocessing steps were applied to the data, and the results showed a considerable improvement in model accuracy. I will discuss the preprocessing techniques and the code in a more readable format. For a better understanding of CT pictures and a relative quantitative measurement of the strength of radio waves, radiologists utilize the HU. During the CT reconstruction process, a grayscale image is created using the radiation absorption/attenuation coefficient within a tissue. The Hounsfield scale that results from the linear translation appears as grey tones on the screen. Less dense tissues have negative values and appear dark; more dense tissues have positive values and appear brighter due to more X-ray beam absorption. HU has been named in honor the illustrious Sir Godfrey Hounsfield, who contributed to the development of CT and received the Nobel Prize in recognition of his work. Using the Rescale Intercept and Rescale Slope headings, we can find the HU.

Since the data is improved after implementation, reducing noises is a crucial part of the preprocessing process. This allows for improved model training. The alignment of the brain image in a suggested manner is called tilt correction. Tilt in brain CT scans may cause misalignment when used for medical purposes. It is crucial because it allows the model to view all of the data uniformly when it is being trained. Manual tilt correction for large-scale data requires significant effort and cost. As a result, tilt correction during preprocessing prior to training needs to be done automatically. Image cropping is required to remove extraneous elements from the image and center the brain image. Additionally, some brain pictures may be positioned differently within the overall image. We need to ensure that almost all of the photographs are in the same location inside the overall image by cropping the image and adding pads.

1.4 MEDICAL IMAGE ANALYSIS

Over time, a multitude of medical image analysis methods have evolved, driven by advancements in artificial neural networks (ANNs) and the continuous progress of deep learning technology. These developments have opened up significant opportunities for highly accurate disease detection across a wide spectrum of X-ray, CT, and MRI images. One of the key technologies enabling this progress is Convolutional Neural Networks[5], often referred to as Conv-Nets or CNNs. CNNs represent a deep learning paradigm that excels in processing input images. They achieve this by assigning importance to various elements and objects within the images through learnable weights and biases, subsequently making fine distinctions between them. Notably, CNNs require considerably less preprocessing compared to alternative classification techniques. They possess the unique capability to autonomously learn filters and features, a stark departure from earlier methods that heavily relied on manually engineered filters.

The architectural design of CNNs draws inspiration from the organization of the human Visual Cortex and closely resembles the intricate network of interconnected neurons found in the brain. In this context, individual neurons respond exclusively within a defined area referred to as the Receptive Field. These fields overlap across the entire visual domain, providing CNNs with a comprehensive coverage that empowers them to effectively process intricate visual information. Research in the field of medical image processing has experienced significant growth over the past few decades [6–8]. Medical imaging has become increasingly crucial in disease diagnosis, driving the exploration of methods based on ANNs. A comprehensive overview of neural networks in image processing was published [9]. One notable challenge in medical image processing is the often-lower signal-to-noise ratio compared to images captured with digital cameras. This reduced signal quality frequently results in lower spatial resolution and diminished contrast between anatomical structures, making accurate computation more challenging. For instance, speckle noise in ultrasonic pictures, which is brought on by the ultrasonic beam's dispersion from tiny tissue in homogeneities, tends to conceal the presence of low contrast lesions and hinders a human observer's capacity to resolve fine detail [10]. Modifications to visual content in the medical field must adhere strict regulations and be carried out in a trustworthy manner that does not compromise clinical judgment. For instance, while it is generally acceptable to eliminate small, bright noise patches, caution is paramount when dealing with mammography to avoid inadvertently removing microcalcifications. Achieving this objective often necessitates the execution of complex operations, with image segmentation playing a pivotal role in the process.

1.5 APPLICATION OF THE GENERATIVE PRE-TRAINED TRANSFORMER (GPT) IN IMAGE ANALYSIS

GPT is a neural network architecture renowned for its exceptional performance in natural language processing tasks. More recently, it has exhibited promising capabilities in image analysis tasks.

The core functionality of the GPT model family relies on the self-attention mechanism and multi-headed attention mechanism, integrated into an encoder-decoder model.

In the realm of image analysis, GPT model serves as a generative tool for creating images resembling those in the training dataset. This is accomplished through initial pre-training on a large image dataset followed by fine-tuning on a smaller, specific image dataset.

- The Vision Transformer (ViT), a GPT variant tailored for image analysis, utilizes self-attention to capture both global and local image features. It segments the input image into patches, flattens each patch into vectors, processes them with self-attention, and finally employs a multi-layer perceptron (MLP) to derive the ultimate image representation.
- One application of the ViT model is image classification, where it predicts image class labels by extracting features with self-attention and employing them for classification.
- The ViT model exhibits significant potential in image analysis and has the capacity to excel in certain tasks when compared to traditional CNNs. However, it remains a relatively new model, necessitating further research to fully comprehend its strengths and limitations.
- CNNs are known for their robustness and relatively easier and quicker training compared to ViT models. ViT model training demands substantial programming effort and can be time-intensive. Moreover, ViT architectures offer limited customization compared to CNNs.

For those interested in medical imagery applications, this book primarily focuses on CNNs, making it accessible even to beginners seeking to clarify concepts.

1.6 HOW TO USE THIS BOOK

The primary target audience of this book comprises undergraduate students, postgraduate students, and researchers interested in exploring medical image analysis using deep learning. The book majorly emphasizes hands-on development rather than only theory-based approach. After studying the theory, readers should practice the sample codes. The platform that has been chosen for this book is Python, which is completely open source, and the packages that have been used for deep learning are also completely open source. The book primarily guides the reader to understand the basic building blocks of deep learning approach and how to use different deep learning models to predict diseases from various types of medical images.

1.7 CONCLUSION

This chapter primarily discusses the evolution of different medical imaging techniques and their background history. The basic building block of medical imaging starts from X-ray. Then it evolved and nowadays digital X-ray comes into picture. Also CT, MRI, and PET scans give ample opportunity to analyze diseases quickly and precisely. The chapters of this book have been organized as follows. Chapter 2 discusses the fundamentals of CNNs. Chapter 3 illustrates the detection of COVID-19 pneumonia using Inception V3 and Custom Designed Bi-Modal Looping DCNN via analysis of X-ray images. Chapter 4 discusses the detection of pneumonia from a small-scale dataset of X-ray images of lungs by using a compound Batch-Normalizing Convolutional Neural Feature Extracting Random Forest Classifier. Chapter 5 describes an adaptive profound transfer learning strategy for malaria cell parasite classification and detection. Chapter 6 implements a Deep Convolutional Auto-Encoding Image-Reconstruction Network to visualize distinct categories of COVID-19 and pneumonia X-ray image features (DCARN). Chapter 7 describes Super Resolution Generative Adversarial Neural Network with Bi-Modal Multi-Perceptron Layers for Medical X-ray Images (SR-GANN), and Chapter 8 concludes the book.

REFERENCES

1. Arfelli, Fulvia, M. Assante, V. Bonvicini, A. Bravin, Giovanni Cantatore, Edoardo Castelli, L. Dalla Palma et al. 2019. Low-dose phase contrast X-ray medical imaging. *Physics in Medicine & Biology*, 43(10), p. 2845.
2. Lundervold, Alexander Selvikvåg, and Arvid Lundervold. 2019. An overview of deep learning in medical imaging focusing on MRI. *Zeitschrift für Medizinische Physik*, 29(2), pp. 102–127.
3. Tahmasebzadeh, Atefeh, Reza Paydar, Mojtaba Soltani-Kermanshahi, Asghar Maziar, and Reza Reiazi. 2021. Lifetime attributable cancer risk related to prevalent CT scan procedures in pediatric medical imaging centers. *International Journal of Radiation Biology*, 97(9), pp. 1282–1288.
4. Venkatesan, C., P. Karthigaikumar, Anand Paul, S. Satheeskumaran, and Rajagopal Kumar. 2018. ECG signal preprocessing and SVM classifier-based abnormality detection in remote healthcare applications. *IEEE Access*, 6, pp. 9767–9773.
5. Ritter, Felix, Tobias Boskamp, André Homeyer, Hendrik Laue, Michael Schwier, Florian Link, and H-O. Peitgen. 2011. Medical image analysis. *IEEE Pulse*, 2(6), pp. 60–70.

6. Doi, Kunio. 2007. Computer-aided diagnosis in medical imaging: Historical review, current status and future potential. *Computerized Medical Imaging and Graphics*, 25(4–5), pp. 198–211.
7. Doi, K. 2005. Current status and future potential of computer-aided diagnosis in medical imaging. *The British Journal of Radiology*, 78, pp. S3–S19.
8. Summers, R.M. 2003. Road maps for advancement of radiologic computer-aided detection in the 21st century. *Radiology*, 229, pp. 11–13.
9. Miller, A.S., B.H. Blott, and T.K. Hames. 1992. Review of neural network applications in medical imaging and signal processing. *Medical & Biological Engineering & Computing*, 30(5), pp. 449–464.
10. Thijssen, Johan M. 2003. Ultrasonic speckle formation, analysis and processing applied to tissue characterization. *Pattern Recognition Letters*, 24(4–5), pp. 659–675.

2 The Convolutional Neural Network

2.1 INTRODUCTION

Images play a vital role in addressing practical challenges. In today's data-driven era, where data volumes are expanding at an unprecedented rate, deep learning has emerged as a key player in solving complex big data problems. Deep learning, a subset of machine learning, harnesses artificial neural networks to tackle data analysis tasks. It finds its applications in various research domains, including computer vision, speech recognition, and natural language processing. Neural networks are central to addressing these real-world challenges. In some cases, neural network designs incorporate convolution operations, leading to systems known as Convolutional Neural Networks (CNNs).

For instance, if the goal is to identify spam websites or emails, one can employ deep learning techniques such as CNNs. CNNs belong to a class of neural networks specifically tailored for visual recognition tasks. They consist of multiple layers known as convolutional layers, designed to focus on distinct detection challenges. CNNs are widely adopted in image processing and pattern recognition, relying on convolution operations to detect key features within images. This enables them to enhance the delineation of objects within images or pinpoint an object's location. To effectively utilize CNNs, selecting appropriate parameters like filters, kernel size, stride size, and padding is essential. In addition, choosing the right architectural configuration for the CNN is crucial. CNNs leverage convolution principles to process images. An image can be envisioned as a numerical matrix comprising three channels: RGB, denoting red, green, and blue channels.

Figure 2.1 illustrates the representation of an image using three distinct color channels. These channels are composed of numerical values that collectively compose the entire image. In the realm of image analysis and processing, the conventional approach involved normalizing these channel matrices to facilitate various complex feature extraction procedures aimed at capturing insights into value distribution. CNN employs the fundamental concept of convolution on these channel matrices. Convolution, in essence, entails the sequential summation of pixel values obtained through simultaneous multiplication of the values within the channel matrix by a designated convolutional kernel. This convolutional kernel is essentially another matrix with predefined dimensions, containing values capable of performing intricate

DOI: 10.1201/9781003456476-2

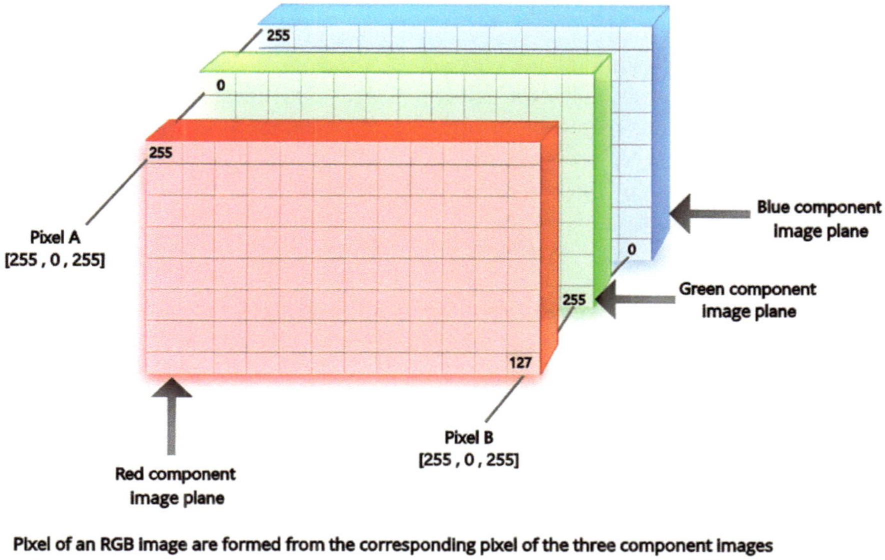

FIGURE 2.1 The diagrammatic representation of a colored RGB image.

tasks such as image edge detection, curvature recognition, identification of pixel value distributions, and many others.

The kernel size is the number of rows and columns in a kernel matrix. The value of a particular pixel in the input image is multiplied by the corresponding value in the kernel matrix and then summed up over all the pixels in the kernel matrix. This sum is then divided by the sum of all the values in the kernel matrix to get the convolutional activation value for that pixel. The effect of a convolutional kernel is to spread the influence of a particular pixel in the input image to some number of adjacent pixels. The number of adjacent pixels whose values are influenced by a particular pixel is called the spatial extent of that kernel.

CNNs are mainly inspired by how the human brain's visual cortex works. According to research done by D.H. Hubel and T.N. Wiesel, CNNs are biologically inspired neural network models. The researchers proposed an awesome explanation for how mammals visually perceive the world around them. This visual perception mechanism was executed by the human brain is a very complex hierarchical way. The visual cortex uses a layered architecture of neurons in the brain, and this, in turn, inspired researchers like us to attempt and develop similar recognition mechanisms in computer vision and deep learning with neural networks.

2.1.1 The Visual Cortex of the Brain

The human brain has two types of neurons: the simple and complex cells. These cells perform different functions in the visual cortex. Simple cells are mainly sensitive to edges, lines, and corners, which correspond to the basic features of the image. Complex cells are sensitive to more complex features like curves, shapes, and patterns. The human visual cortex is structured into six layers of neurons with various functions. Each layer within the network serves a specific hierarchical function. The initial layer's neurons specialize in detecting edges and lines, while those in subsequent layers generate increasingly intricate representations of the input image. Ultimately, the final layer produces an output that is recognizable to an observer. CNNs are organized into layers, each with roles akin to those in the human cortex. The output of one layer serves as input for the next, with each layer working toward crafting more intricate image representations. The ultimate layer produces a classification for the input image.

Neural networks constitute complex systems of interconnected neurons and have proven invaluable in solving various machine learning challenges. A key advantage of neural networks is their capacity to learn from data, eliminating the need for predefined rules. Instead, they undergo a "learning" or "training" phase where they discern patterns within input data and classify it accordingly. During the subsequent "testing" phase, they apply these learned patterns to classify new inputs. If errors occur, they can be corrected, leading to further training and performance enhancement. Neural networks comprise neurons, which can vary in complexity, and these neurons are organized into layers. Each neuron in one layer is connected to every neuron in the next layer, facilitating the flow of information throughout the network.

So, there will be one input layer, one output layer, and one or more hidden layers in between. The input layer takes input data and transforms it into signals which can be understood by the network. The output layer transforms these signals into a form that can be interpreted by an outside observer. Hidden layers in between transform these signals from simple to complex and vice versa. The process of training the neural network is called the "training" phase. In this step, we need to give inputs with their corresponding outputs to the network for learning. One way to do this is to give all the training data for the network and then let the network run. Once it is done, the network will have learned the pattern from the training data and will be ready for testing. In the testing phase, we give some inputs which are not part of the training data. We expect that the network will classify them correctly. If it does, then we can say that the network has learned well and it will be ready for deployment. Thus, within the visual cortex, complex functional responses are generated by very complex cells that are constructed from more responses from simple cells. For instance, the simple cells would always respond to the oriented edges of the images, while the complex cells will also respond to oriented edges but with a varying degree of spatial in-variances.

In the primary visual cortex (V1), more complex cells respond to stimuli that are more complex in nature. For instance, these complex cells will respond to two lines at an angle of 30 degrees with a slight offset, while simple cells in V1 will respond to either one line or two parallel lines. Thus, the neurons in V1 respond to the orientation of the lines but the complex cells will also respond to the angle of the lines. Complex cells in higher areas of the visual association cortex can also respond to multiple stimulus attributes such as color, size, location, and movement. The process of visual perception involves a series of stages that lead from raw sensory information to a subjective experience. This process is known as perception and is a fundamental cognitive process. Perception is possible through the process of sensory transduction and synaptic transmission. Sensory transduction converts physical energy into neural signals. The neural signals are then transmitted through neurons to the synaptic terminal, which interacts with other neurons at the synaptic level. These interactions result in a series of stages that allow an individual to perceive visual stimuli. Perception is a highly complex and dynamic process. For instance, during visual perception, the visual system (eyes and brain) must be able to maintain a clear image despite the fact that the image is constantly changing due to external factors such as movement and illumination changes. This task is accomplished by using different types of neurons that can maintain a specific threshold of activity regardless of the external factors. Further, perception involves the integration of multiple sensory modalities. For instance, in the visual system, information from the visual, auditory, and somatosensory systems is integrated to form a singular experience. Finally, perception involves the ability to recognize objects and interpret their meaning. For instance, an individual can see a picture of a face but must be able to recognize that this face is a representation of a human being.

The "perceptron" model, introduced by psychologist Frank Rosenblatt in 1958, marked the first attempt to create a computational model of how the brain processes visual information for perception. The perceptron was conceptualized as a large switch capable of carrying out pattern recognition tasks. It serves as a straightforward linear classifier comprising three essential layers: the input layer, the output layer, and an intermediary layer. The input layer mirrors the sensory receptors of the visual system, akin to the eyes and optic nerve. The output layer, referred to as "dendrites," generates a single-bit output based on the input received. In between lies the "hidden layer," responsible for receiving input from the input layer, processing these inputs, and generating activation values (activation maps) that play a crucial role in determining the final output. The operation of the visual cortex and the human brain can be explained through the concept of receptive fields, where individual cells respond to the summation of inputs from neighboring cells. Deep CNNs draw inspiration from these ideas. They utilize local connections to link each component in a hierarchical manner. This layering approach ensures that data follows a hierarchical path, enabling the recognition of specific faces or images under varying conditions. This is achieved through the acquisition of abstractions that are invariant to changes in size, contrast, rotation, orientation, and other factors, resulting in a robust recognition system.

2.2 ADVANCEMENTS IN THE FIELD OF DEEP LEARNING AND CONVOLUTIONAL NEURAL NETWORKS

A perceptron serves as the foundational building block for constructing a deep neural network. Essentially, a perceptron is a single-layer neural network that takes input and produces a linear response. The output is determined by the neuron with the highest activation level, effectively becoming the overall output. To refine the perceptron's output, a logistic function is typically applied after the linear function. This logistic function, often referred to as the "sigmoid function," scales the linear output to a value between 0 and 1. Comparatively, when evaluating the output of a single neuron versus a perceptron, the linear function is followed by the sigmoid function. A deep neural network is formed by connecting numerous perceptrons across multiple layers. Each layer receives inputs from the preceding layer and generates outputs, which are subsequently transmitted to the subsequent layer. This process continues until the final layer produces an output that is compared with the desired target output.

In general, neural networks consist of neurons organized into multiple layers. Neurons are interconnected within the same layer and with neurons in subsequent layers. The training of neural networks typically employs supervised learning algorithms, which instruct the network to generate the correct output for any given input by utilizing a set of input patterns alongside their corresponding desired outputs. During this process, known as forward propagation, the neural network's weights and thresholds (referred to as parameters) are adjusted until it can accurately produce the correct response for each training pattern. To fine-tune the neural network's weights and thresholds, a backpropagation algorithm is utilized. A "link" represents a connection between two nodes within the network, and the weight assigned to this connection is known as the "connection weight." The advantage of using a gradient descent scheme is that it allows for local adjustments to the network parameters, which may reduce the risk of over-adjusting the parameters. Deep neural networks have been applied to many problem domains, such as computer vision, speech recognition, and natural language processing. They have also been applied to problems such as game playing (e.g., chess and Japanese Go game), medical diagnosis, machine translation, social network filtering, predicting stock prices, and climate modeling. The first working deep neural network was published by Alexey Grigorevich Ivakhnenko and V. G. Lapa in 1965. This network had two layers of neurons – an input layer and an output layer. The input layer had five neurons, which received inputs from a single sensor that represented a binary input. The output layer contained two neurons, one of which represented a "yes" answer and the other represented a "no" answer.

Rosenblatt created the first deep neural network in the Western world in 1958. He called it a perceptron, and it had three layers: an input layer, a middle layer, and an output layer. The network had 2 neurons in the input layer, 20 neurons in the middle layer, and 1 neuron in the output layer. The middle layer neurons were connected to the input layer neurons and the output layer neuron. The perceptron was trained to classify patterns from binary inputs. It classified patterns as either 1 or 2. In 1969, Widrow and Hoff improved the model by replacing the binary inputs with the real-valued inputs and adding a learning rule. With this modification, their model could learn how to adjust its weights to correctly classify a wide variety of patterns. Deep neural networks found their first successes in the early 1990s when they began to be applied to recognizing hand-written digits and other tasks that require very large labeled training sets. Deep learning started becoming popular after the publication of a landmark paper in *Nature* by Hinton, Osindero, and the, published in the year of 2006. This paper introduced a deep autoencoder that used unsupervised pre-training to bootstrap the learning of a deep network. The unsupervised pre-training helped the network overcome the vanishing gradient problem. The paper also demonstrated the advantages of deep learning over other machine learning methods on a handwriting recognition task. In 2006, a team of researchers from the University of Toronto, including Geoffrey Hinton, published a paper in the journal *Science* that demonstrated how a deep neural network could be trained to map images to precise locations in 3D space using the location of the human eyes as an input. In 2012, Li Deng and his colleagues at Stanford published the first real-time object detection system based on deep learning. Their work used a large number of deep filters (over 5 million) and was able to detect multiple objects in a scene with a high level of precision and recall. In 2014, a team of researchers from Google led by Andrew Ng published a paper that described a deep learning method for relabeling optical flow. Their method outperformed the previous state-of-the-art system for optical flow estimation on the Oxford Flowers data set. In 2014, DeepMind unveiled a groundbreaking achievement in the field of artificial intelligence (AI) through a paper detailing an AI system that independently learned to master Atari games without any human intervention. The AI was trained with a reward-based system, earning points for performing well in the games and losing points for errors. Over thousands of self-played games, it progressively honed its gaming abilities. After mastering video games, it went on to defeat professional human players at "Space Invaders."

During the same year, Google introduced the Inception V3, an advanced algorithm designed for image recognition. The primary aim was to delve deeper into convolutional techniques and surpass existing state-of-the-art algorithms. Moving on to 2015, Google's Auto-ML initiative, focused on automating the creation of deep neural networks, demonstrated significant progress by halving the error rates of the networks it generated. In parallel, Microsoft researchers, including Xiaolong Wang, delved into applying deep learning to the complex realm of protein folding. Their pioneering work resulted in the development of a neural network capable of achieving near-human-level accuracy. This achievement was realized by utilizing a neural network to analyze the atomic structure of proteins and predict their functions based on their structural characteristics.

2.3 IMPLEMENTATION OF A BASIC CONVOLUTIONAL NEURAL NETWORK USING PYTHON AND TENSORFLOW

A. Conv2D

The Conv2D class is one of the few classes in Keras that has its constructor, and it accepts several arguments. It is used to perform a two-dimensional convolution based on a set of weights and filters. The filters can be 3×3 or 5×5 sized and this class will also accept padding values of "same," "valid," or "same".

B. Max Pooling2D

The MaxPooling2D class is responsible for conducting a pooling operation on a tensor. This pooling operation offers various configuration options, primarily governed by the pool_size, strides, and padding arguments. Pooling serves the purpose of reducing the volume of parameters that require learning within the model.

For instance, if we initially have an input volume sized at [5, 5, 100], following the pooling operation, its dimensions become [5, 5, 30]. This transformation effectively diminishes the number of model parameters that need to be learned. Pooling brings multiple advantages, including a reduction in computational complexity and an enhancement in the model's processing speed. Consequently, it is highly advisable to incorporate pooling techniques during the training of a neural network.

C. **Spatial Convolution**
The Spatial Convolution class is used to perform a convolution with the given weights and filters, but here instead of using a two-dimensional filter, we are passing a one-dimensional filter to it. The filter shape must be a tuple containing an integer for the number of channels in the input and an integer for the number of outputs in the output volume.

D. **Max Pooling1D**
The MaxPooling1D class performs a one-dimensional pooling operation on a tensor. The pool_size argument configures the pooling operation. This class reduces the size of the input volume by a factor equal to the pool_size. That is why it reduces the number of parameters that need to be learned by the model. Pooling also helps in reducing computational cost and enhances the speed of the model. Thus, it is recommended to use pooling while training the network.

E. **Dropout Layer**
This layer is used to reduce the number of connections between the input and output layers. It is a feed-forward layer with a single neuron. When training starts, we randomly assign a set of neurons to be turned off (i.e. their outputs are zero). Then, we wait for a few iterations, to see if the error rate is decreasing; if it isn't, we change the neurons that are turned off. This procedure continues until the error rate is low enough.

Figure 2.2 illustrates a CNN engaged in the task of multi-class image classification, specifically using the well-known MNIST digits dataset. This dataset contains various images of handwritten digits. The network's initial layer is referred to as the Input Layer, where inputs are resized to a specified dimension of 28×28×1. This means that the image has a height and width of 28 pixels, with a single-color channel.

Moving forward, the first convolutional layer (Conv_1) comes into play. It conducts convolution operations utilizing a predefined number of convolution kernels, each with a size of 5×5, while also applying valid padding to the images. Following this initial convolution, the input image, originally sized at 28×28×1, transforms into 24×24×N1, where N1 represents the number of convolution kernels or feature maps. This operation simultaneously reduces the image size and increases the number of feature maps. Subsequently, the max pooling layer enters the picture, tasked with capturing a fixed pixel distribution from the resulting convolutional feature maps. The input for this max pooling layer is derived from the output of the first convolutional layer, having dimensions of 24×24×N1. After executing a 2×2 max pooling operation, the size of the convolutional output tensor becomes 12×12×N1. This process reduces image size while maintaining a constant feature map vector (N1). Once the max pooling step is successfully completed, the outputs are forwarded to the next convolutional layer, denoted as Conv_2. This layer employs an approach similar to the first convolution layer, using N2 kernels with dimensions of 5×5, and applies valid padding for improved image optimization. The output from the max pooling layer, originally sized at 12×12×N1, transforms into 8×8×N2 within the second convolutional layer.

Thus, further the height and width of the images are reduced but the value of N2 is generally kept more than N1 for better feature capturing. Generally, during real-time applications, the values of N1 and N2 are 64 and 128, respectively, depending on the complexity of the images. Thus, the output of the Conv_2 layer is fed to the

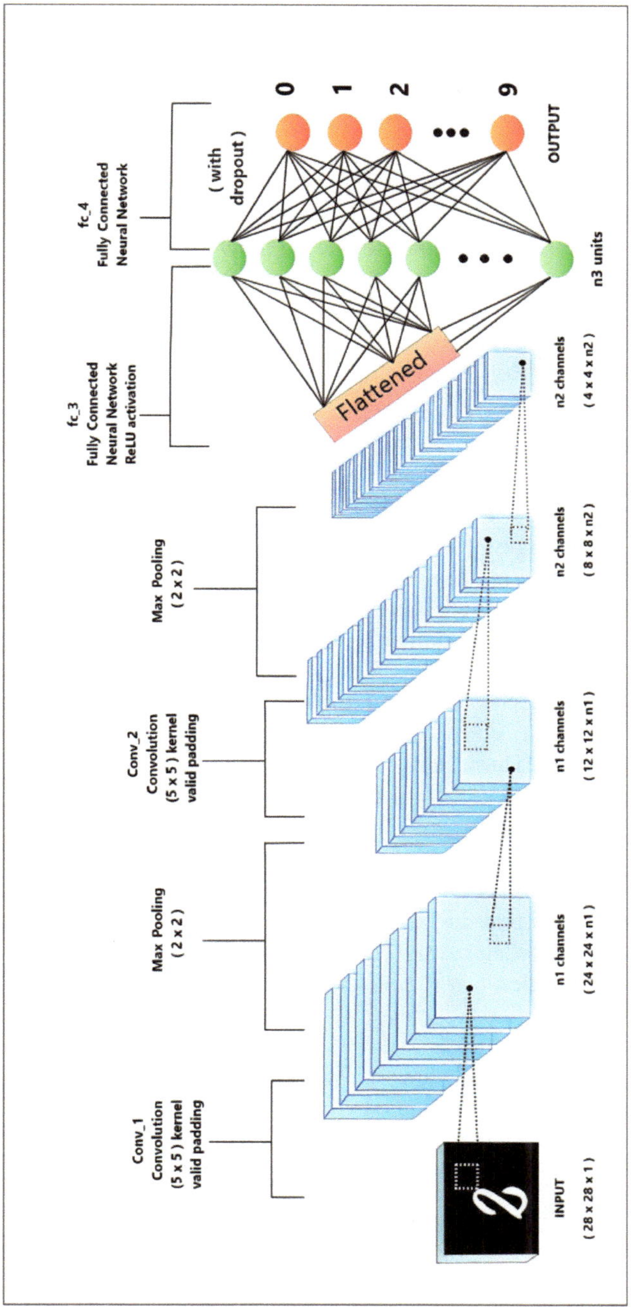

FIGURE 2.2 A pictorial representation of a convolutional neural network for multi-class classification.

second max pooling layer for assuring further reduction of the outputs of the second convolution layer. The max pooling layer again uses the same principle of height and width reduction but keeps the number of feature matrices the same as N2. Thus, as mentioned above, the size of the second max pooling feature matrix was 2×2, and hence the output of the max pooling layer was 4×4×N2. Finally, since we are dealing with CNNs, the output of the max pooling layer was multiplied with each other, like 4×4×N2. Let the value of N2 be 128 as mentioned earlier, then the output of the flatten layer which is applied after the second max pooling layer will be 2048. The fully connected (fc_3) is the main artificial neural network that has been applied to the outputs of the flattening layer, justified with the N3 number of hidden neurons that use the rectified linear activation function. N3 can be replaced with 2048 and, finally, the ultimate layer, fc_4, acts as the output layer of the entire CNN and has only ten hidden neurons with softmax activation for performing the required multi-class classification.

2.4 TRANSFER LEARNING IN CONVOLUTIONAL NEURAL NETWORKS

2.4.1 Introduction about Transfer Learning

In deep learning, the main problem that researchers face is the problem of computation resources. The models in deep learning, especially CNNs, are computationally quite expensive. In order to allow researchers to incorporate sophisticated models of deep learning into their specific domain problems, the concept of transfer learning plays an important role, as explained by Torrey et al. [1] and Pan et al. [2]. In transfer learning, the main objective is to use the already trained and designed neural network models, like Inception V3 by Google or VGG16 by Visual Graphics Group, for our domain-specific tasks. These state-of-the-art algorithms are quite capable of capturing image-related features, as these networks were trained on millions and millions of images. Utilizing these powers and learned features in a perfect way can help solve image recognition, image classification, and image feature capturing, as explained by Long et al. [3] and Ravishankar et al. [4].

Transfer learning is comprised of two different segments. One is called fine-tuning, where we use pre-trained models to train our models. For example, we have a pre-trained model for image classification that is quite good. We can use it to fine-tune our model for image recognition in order to increase its performance. The other part of transfer learning is where we take our model and retrain it using a new dataset. We retrain the model by feeding it the new dataset and by using the pre-trained models to classify the new dataset. This training of the existing state-of-art algorithms on our custom dataset is known as the pre-training of the neural networks. In certain applications, we even train the existing neural networks from scratch, as we need not design the former.

2.4.2 Some of the Famous Transfer Learning Examples of Convolutional Neural Network

2.4.2.1 Inception V3 aka GoogLeNet

The diagram provided in Figure 2.3 may seem intricate at first glance, but upon closer examination, one can decipher its structure. This image represents the sophisticated

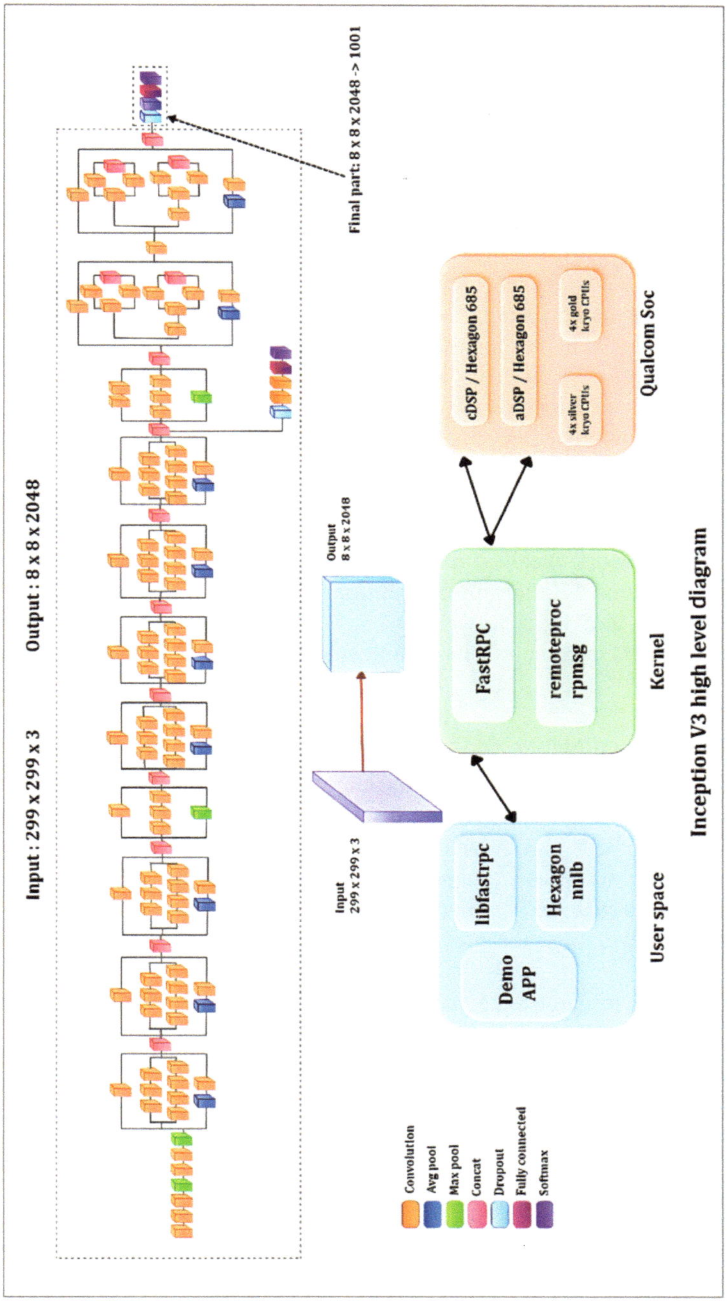

FIGURE 2.3 The Inception V3 architecture as designed by Google in 2014.

Inception V3 model, as introduced by Szegedy et al. [5] in 2014, for image recognition and classification, developed by Google.

This neural network, known as Inception V3, is a CNN featuring over 100 convolution and max pooling layers applied at various stages in unique configurations. The key innovation behind the inception network lies in its adoption of asymmetrical convolutions, departing from the conventional symmetrical convolutions utilized by Mollahosseini et al. [6]. This strategic shift brings about several advantages, including a reduction in the number of required filters. Additionally, it enhances the amount of retained information within the network, ultimately boosting recognition accuracy.

Inception V3 is proficient in classifying images into a wide range of 1,000 distinct categories. The network comprises a total of six layers, with the first five layers featuring 64 nodes each and the final layer containing 1,000 nodes. These categories are further divided into classes. This network achieves image classification by internalizing representations of images through training. The training process employs an error backpropagation algorithm, where a set of images is classified into each of the 1,000 categories.

Inception V3's remarkable capabilities extend to recognizing objects within natural images. It leverages the architecture of CNNs to extract features essential for recognition. The network excels at recognizing objects across varying scales, poses, and lighting conditions. Furthermore, Inception V3 can identify objects in the form of text, handwriting, and digits, as well as shapes and images. Its versatility in recognizing diverse objects underscores its significance in the realm of image recognition and classification.

2.4.2.2 The Residual Network Architecture (aka ResNet-50)

Another interesting application of transfer learning is using the Residual Network learning proposed by Kaiming He in his research paper, "Deep Residual Learning." The main concept of this particular model is the incorporation of skip connections in between internal layers, as explained by He et al. [7]. This particular model is a variant of the traditional Resnet model, which uses residual connections between the convolutional layers and the previous layers (or the output layers in traditional Resnet).

The authors of the research paper have claimed that this particular model overcomes the major limitation of the traditional Resnet model, which is under-fitting. Although this model is highly beneficial, further research is still being carried out to adopt this model in a real-world scenario.

The major limitation of this model lies in the size of the network, which increases exponentially as more layers are added to the network, as Wei et al. [8] explain. This model is, however, a popular choice in transfer learning because it is not only computationally efficient but also has a very high performance.

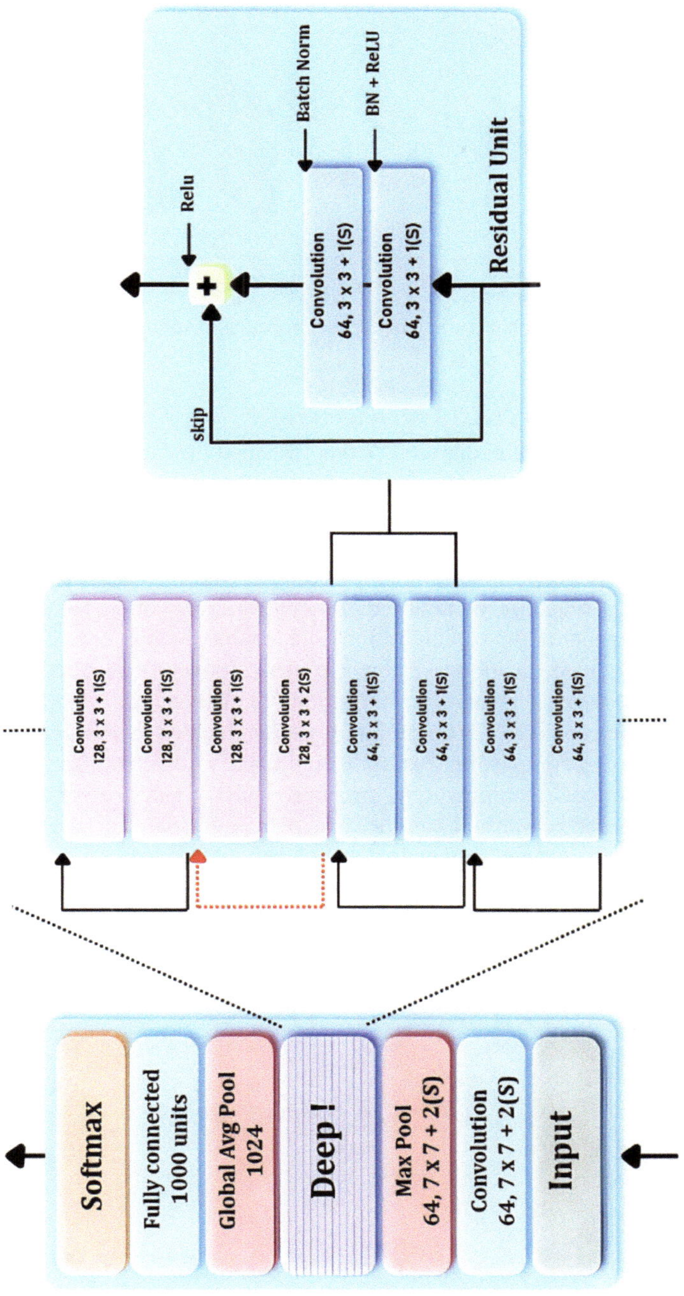

FIGURE 2.4 The main concept of residual networks is depicted.

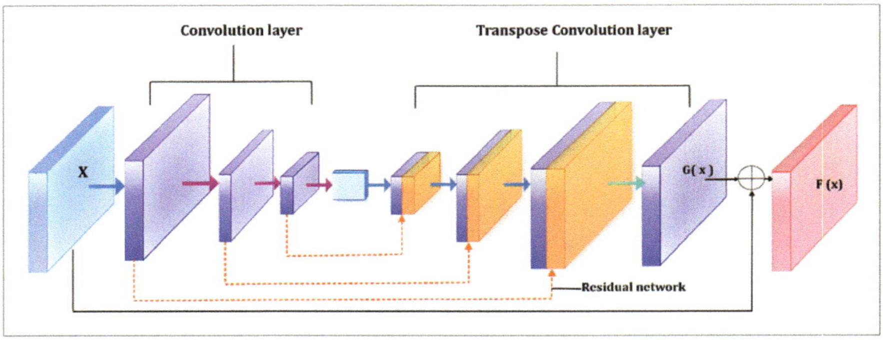

FIGURE 2.5 The ResNet architecture with the mentioned skip connections.

2.4.2.3 The VGG16 and VGG19 Architecture

VGG16 stands out as a revolutionary CNN that reshaped the landscape of image processing within the research community. Its landmark achievement was being the first layered CNN to achieve top rankings in the ImageNet competition, an accomplishment attributed to Simonyan et al. [9]. Proposed by the Visual Graphics Group (VGG), VGG16 marked a significant milestone in the realm of multi-class image recognition. The model boasts a sequence of multiple consecutive convolutional layers, meticulously designed to enhance the capture of intricate features within input images. What sets VGG16 apart is its dedication to using symmetric convolutions, in contrast to the asymmetrical convolutions favored by Inception V3. Efficiency, effectiveness, and robustness are at the core of VGG16's design. It was engineered to deliver superior performance in processing complex images while optimizing resource utilization, reducing both parameter count and computational demands. VGG16 offers a versatile balance between computational power and memory usage, making it a preferred choice for a broad spectrum of projects and applications, much like the work of Santos et al. [10].

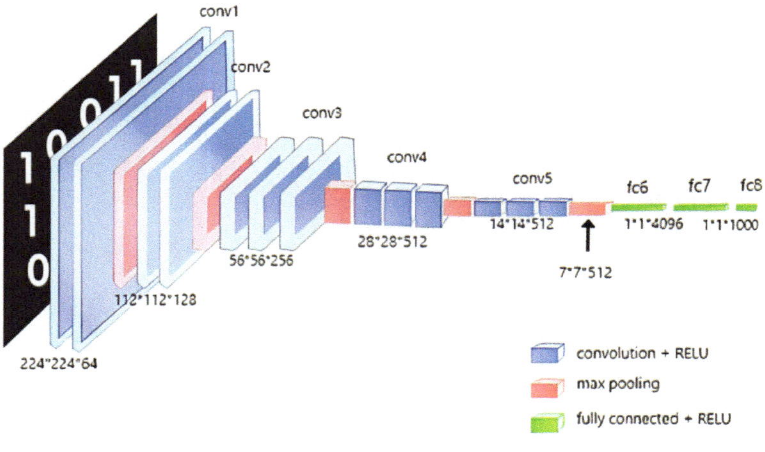

FIGURE 2.6 The VGG16 architecture for custom class classification.

Figure 2.6 shows the VGG16 architecture. The model is comprised of six convolutional layers, max-pooling layers, batch normalization layers, and ReLU units. The VGG16 is the first CNN that was used in the ImageNet competition. VGG16 was designed to be a very strong model that would also be very easy to use. It is quite effective even though it has a lightweight structure. This model was developed to be quite robust and effective in terms of computing power, memory usage, and training speed. It was designed to be new and efficient and also to be a very robust model that could solve the problems found in the previous models. The model was designed to be robust and effective and also be very easy to use. Complex models like Auto-Encoders and Variational Auto-Encoders use these architectures for the encoder and decoder designs.

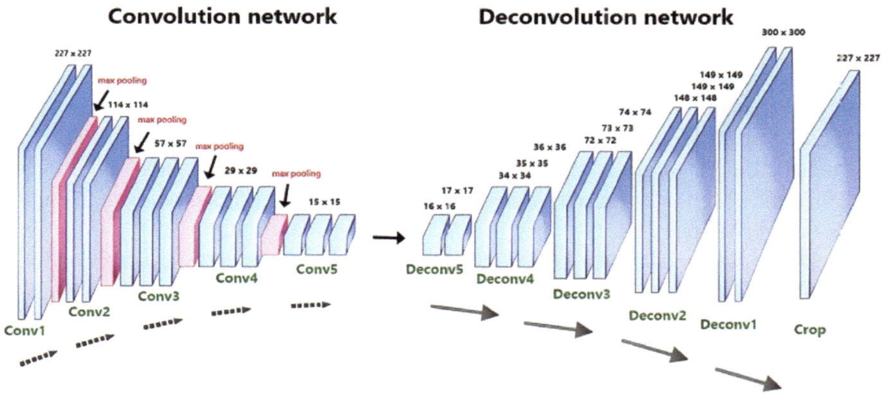

FIGURE 2.7 An auto-encoder using VGG16 state-of-the-art transfer learning.

2.5 A COMPARATIVE STUDY BETWEEN ADVANCED CNN SYSTEMS, GENERATIVE ADVERSARIAL NEURAL NETWORK (GANN), AND STABLE DIFFUSION (SD) MODEL

Generative adversarial networks (GANs) and SD are two popular approaches used for image generation. While both techniques can generate high-quality images, they differ in terms of their underlying architecture and training methods.

GANs are primarily composed of two neural networks: a generator and a discriminator.

- The generator takes a random noise vector as input and generates an image, while the discriminator takes an image as input and determines whether it is real or fake. The two networks are trained together in a min-max game, where the generator tries to generate realistic images to fool the discriminator, and the discriminator tries to correctly identify real images from the generated ones. This iterative process of training leads to the generator learning to produce increasingly realistic images.

SD, on the other hand, is a continuous diffusion process that generates images by iteratively adding Gaussian noise to an initial image.

- In each iteration, the noise level is increased, and the image is updated using a partial differential equation. The process is repeated multiple times until the desired level of noise is reached, and the final image is obtained. The diffusion process is designed to be stable and ensures that the generated images are coherent and realistic.

In terms of image generation quality, both GANs and SD demonstrate the ability to create high-quality images characterized by realistic textures and intricate details. However, there are nuanced distinctions in the output they produce. GANs tend to yield sharper and more precisely defined images, while SD excels in generating smoother, more lifelike images characterized by natural variations and textures. When it comes to the training aspect, GANs are notorious for their complexity and demand for substantial data volumes to yield satisfactory results. The training process can be prone to instability, necessitating meticulous hyperparameter tuning. On the other hand, SD offers a comparatively simpler training process that requires less data. It requires fewer hyperparameters to fine-tune and exhibits greater resilience to initialization challenges.

Another notable disparity between these approaches pertains to interpretability. GANs often face criticism for their "black-box" nature, as comprehending the inner workings of the generator network can be perplexing. In contrast, SD takes a more interpretable route, as the diffusion process can be visualized and subjected to analysis. To sum it up, GANs and SD stand as two prominent methods for image generation, each with its distinct strengths and weaknesses. GANs excel in producing sharper, more well-defined images but entail a more intricate training process and offer less interpretability. On the other hand, SD thrives in generating smoother, more realistic images, is easier to train, and facilitates greater interpretability. The selection between the two depends on the specific needs of the application and the available resources. In this book, we delve into a particular application, addressing a specific image challenge—super resolution—utilizing a specialized variant of GANs known as the super-resolution GANN.

2.6 CONCLUSION

Deep learning proves to be a powerful tool for addressing various real-world challenges, particularly in the face of exponentially growing datasets. Deep learning algorithms are customarily applied to domain-specific tasks that demand automation and intelligent sensing capabilities. CNNs hold significant value when there is an ample dataset available for training. Often, deep neural network systems undergo optimization procedures to enhance their output quality, ensuring superior results. Researchers have successfully harnessed the capabilities of deep learning, including CNNs, artificial neural networks, recurrent neural networks, long short-term memory networks, and more, to tackle domain-specific issues through the concept of transfer learning. Consequently, when dealing with a vast volume of images, employing CNNs can prove to be highly advantageous.

Transfer learning, although a well-established concept today, has roots dating back to the 1980s in the field of computer vision. Pioneers like Poggio and colleagues independently developed domain adaptation techniques in 1985, enabling the learning of domain-specific feature detectors from data and their application in different domains, such as edge detection and letter recognition. In 1986, Fahlman and colleagues proposed cross-domain learning, which involved transferring knowledge from one problem to another, allowing the solution of a second problem after learning the first. This approach, too, found application in computer vision.

Fast-forward to the early 2000s, when the concept of training deep neural networks with extensive datasets emerged. By 2006, the notion of generalization in neural networks was established, paving the way for advanced applications. In 2009, transfer learning using large datasets gained prominence. Transfer learning serves various objectives. At times, the goal is to enhance model accuracy, while in other scenarios, the focus shifts to reducing model size and improving efficiency, even at the cost of some accuracy.

Multiple methodologies exist for implementing transfer learning, with the following being among the most common:

- Retraining from Scratch: This approach involves retraining a model entirely using a new dataset to boost its performance on a target task. The new dataset often contains richer information compared to the original dataset used for model training.
- Fine-tuning: In this method, an already trained model is fine-tuned on a new dataset, usually by adjusting certain layers or parameters. Fine-tuning is often employed when the original model shares some similarities with the target task.

Transfer learning continues to be a dynamic and evolving field, with diverse strategies and objectives tailored to specific applications and requirements. This approach is suitable for situations where the new dataset has more information than the old dataset. The second approach (fine-tune) is used when one wants to improve the performance of the model on the target task without retraining the model from scratch. In this approach, we use the weights of the model that was already trained on the old dataset. Weights are the parameters of a model that are used to adjust the model weights to give it a particular desired output. In this approach, the weights are used to adjust the model to ensure that the model achieves a better performance on the target task. The model is fine-tuned by adjusting the weights of the model. The advantage of this approach is that it does not require a lot of data to train the model. The disadvantage of this approach is that the model may not achieve the same level of performance as the model that was retrained from scratch.

REFERENCES

1. Torrey, L. and Shavlik, J., 2010. Transfer learning. In *Handbook of research on machine learning applications and trends: Algorithms, methods, and techniques* (pp. 242–264).

2. Pan, S.J. and Yang, Q., 2009. A survey on transfer learning. *IEEE Transactions on Knowledge and Data Engineering*, 22(10), pp. 1345–1359.
3. Long, M., Zhu, H., Wang, J. and Jordan, M.I., 2017. Deep transfer learning with joint adaptation networks. In *International conference on machine learning* (pp. 2208–2217).
4. Ravishankar, H., Sudhakar, P., Venkataramani, R., Thiruvenkadam, S., Annangi, P., Babu, N., and Vaidya, V., 2016. Understanding the mechanisms of deep transfer learning for medical images. In *Deep learning and data labeling for medical applications* (pp. 188–196). Cham: Springer.
5 Szegedy, C., Liu, W., Jia, Y., Sermanet, P., Reed, S., Anguelov, D., Erhan, D., Vanhoucke, V. and Rabinovich, A., 2015. Going deeper with convolutions. In *Proceedings of the IEEE conference on computer vision and pattern recognition.*
6. Mollahosseini, A., Chan, D. and Mahoor, M.H., 2016, March. Going deeper in facial expression recognition using deep neural networks. In *2016 IEEE winter conference on applications of computer vision (WACV)* (pp. 1–10).
7. He, K., Zhang, X., Ren, S. and Sun, J., 2016. Deep residual learning for image recognition. In *Proceedings of the IEEE conference on computer vision and pattern recognition.*
8. Wei, Y., Yuan, Q., Shen, H. and Zhang, L., 2017. Boosting the accuracy of multispectral image pansharpening by learning a deep residual network. *IEEE Geoscience and Remote Sensing Letters*, 14(10), pp. 1795–1799.
9. Simonyan, K. and Zisserman, A., 2014. Very deep convolutional networks for large-scale image recognition. *arXiv preprint arXiv*:1409.1556.
10. Santos, A.G., de Souza, C.O., Zanchettin, C., Macedo, D., Oliveira, A.L. and Ludermir, T., 2018, July. Reducing squeezenet storage size with depthwise separable convolutions. In *2018 International joint conference on neural networks (IJCNN)* (pp. 1–6).

3 The Detection of COVID-19 Pneumonia Using Inception V3 and Custom Designed Bi-Modal Looping DCNN via Analysis of X-Ray Images

3.1 INTRODUCTION

In the realm of medical research and technology, data assumes a pivotal role in addressing real-world challenges. As clinical data continues to accumulate, the imperative to maximize its utility becomes increasingly apparent. Enhancing the size and quality of patient databases stands as a crucial stride toward aiding researchers in discovering solutions. The HealthDataX (HDX) project represents a significant advancement in data management and exchange within the medical domain, particularly for facilitating data sharing in academic research. Leveraging blockchain technology in tandem with smart contracts, HDX introduces a transparent and secure service. Notably, data integrity is guaranteed, as it resides on an immutable public blockchain. This safeguards against tampering, ensuring that any data loss or breach is readily detectable. The implementation of transfer learning and ensemble learning assumes a pivotal role in our work involving chest X-ray classification for the detection of COVID-19. In Figure 3.1 you will find some sample images that we will be addressing as part of this endeavor.

From Figure 3.1 it is clear that at the first glance, differences between the two X-rays could not be identified. The X-ray on the left of Figure 3.1 is of a patient who has not been affected by COVID-19 pneumonia. On the other hand, the picture at the right of Figure 3.1 is of a patient who has been affected by COVID-19 pneumonia. With our naked eye, we cannot determine which of the image is having pneumonia, unless they are labeled. In this chapter, we'll be working with a dataset comprising approximately 5,000 X-ray images depicting COVID-19 pneumonia cases and 3,000 images of normal lung X-rays. These images are labeled and are available in both JPEG and

DOI: 10.1201/9781003456476-3

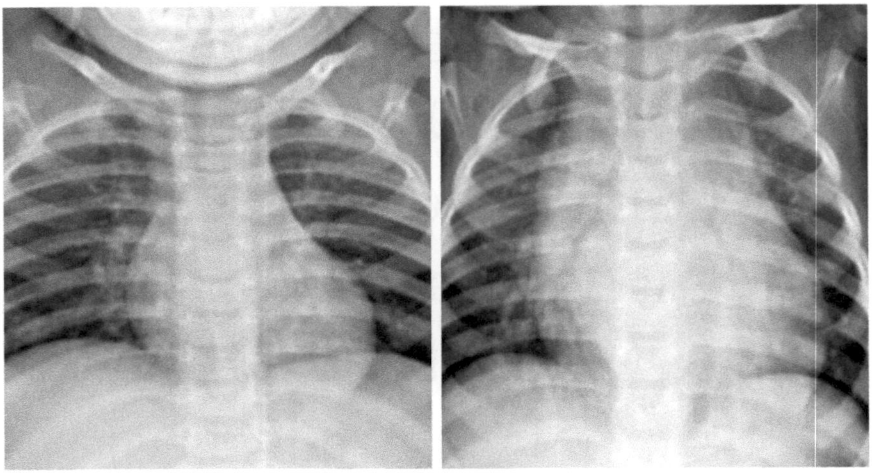

FIGURE 3.1 The normal lung X-ray image (left) and COVID-19 viral pneumonia image (right).

PNG formats. When dealing with high-quality images on such a large scale, the primary algorithm of choice is Deep Convolutional Neural Networks (DCNNs).

In this chapter, we will delve into a comprehensive analysis of these lung X-ray images to tackle the challenges of COVID-19 pneumonia detection. To achieve this, we will employ an exceptional state-of-the-art convolutional neural network (CNN) known as Inception V3. Additionally, we will utilize a complementary network that we've referred to as the Bi-Modal Looping DCNN. This designed system represents an ensemble approach, integrating the capabilities of these two aforementioned CNNs through deep transfer learning techniques.

3.2 RELATED RESEARCH

CNNs play a pivotal role in the field of image classification and can surpass other cutting-edge algorithms in terms of performance [1]. In the realm of medical research and technology, there exists a wealth of opportunities to leverage well-designed systems incorporating deep CNNs [2, 3]. Historically, researchers attempted to address image processing tasks using conventional image processing algorithms, which, although sometimes accurate, fell short of solving specific targeted tasks [4]. Recent advancements, as outlined by Suzuki [3], have demonstrated the potential of deep learning in medical imaging systems, particularly in automating radiologist tasks. The storage of high-quality images for future reference offers the potential to develop sophisticated and accurate data control systems with the assistance of neural networks [5, 6]. Utilizing images from various medical domains to address specific tasks can greatly facilitate automation in medical research. It's worth noting that medical images are highly confidential and exhibit an exceptional level of accuracy, often exceeding 98%. With the advent of advanced imaging devices in hospitals, such as X-ray machines, there has been a significant improvement in the quality of captured images, enabling a wide range of high-end image processing tasks [7–9].

CNNs stand as the cornerstone of deep learning, effectively replacing traditional image processing algorithms through their application of vector and matrix mathematics to images at a sophisticated level. While they are often referred to as "Black Boxes" due to their complex internal operations, they excel at handling image data. However, the effectiveness of deep learning hinges on the exponential growth in the volume of data being processed and the maintenance of data quality. Various medical tests, including X-rays, CT scans, and histopathology, generate a wealth of images that can be stored for future use and automation in decision-making processes [10–12].

Pathologists and doctors can leverage these sophisticated automation systems to enhance the accuracy of their decisions, contributing to a healthier world. Data management and maintenance will continue to be instrumental in shaping the way deep CNNs function, fostering innovation in medical research and technology.

3.3 DATASET DESCRIPTION AND PROGRAMMING LIBRARIES OVERVIEW

In this work, the dataset that we are going to use is composed of basically two different categories of images: normal lung X-ray and COVID-pneumonia lung X-ray. There were originally 5,000 raw images of COVID-pneumonia lung X-rays and 3,000 raw images of normal lung X-rays. Inception V3 is the first component that will be working upon the images along with its support, the Bi-Modal Looping DCNN. Inception V3 would be trained by the image data and the size of the images was increased to a dimension of 300×300×3, height and width being 300 and as colored RGB image so the channels are also 3. The images may be looking like black and white images but they are not, rather X-rays output grey-colored images which can be treated as colored images. The size of the training tensor for the Inception V3 network was kept constant to a value of [4500, 300, 300, 3], where 4500 refers to the total number of images for training and 300, 300, 3 represents the dimension of a single image. The validation data tensor for the Inception V3 network was [300, 300, 300, 3], where 300 refers to a total number of validation images during the training validation step. Finally, the testing tensor was kept constant at [200, 300, 300, 3], where 200 refers to final testing images which the Inception V3 network has not seen earlier. On the other hand, the Bi-Modal Looping DCNN was designed in such a way that it can work with the same dimensions of data tensors as per Inception V3, and thus, the data engineering and processing was completed. The Inception V3 has around 20 million (M) parameters for training and on the other hand, Bi-Modal Looping DCNN has around 10M parameters to train, making the entire system stable and robust.

The entire data preprocessing has been done in Python 3.7 with the help of TensorFlow, OpenCV-Python, and Scikit-Learn. Tensorflow was the main library for the designing of the proposed system and it also helped us to perform some in situ image augmentations to ensure smooth training. Image resizing was conducted with the help of OpenCV and thus, finally, the training and optimization of the ensemble CNN system is also executed using Tensorflow, Tensorboard, and Matplotlib. Performance metrics of the two individual models are also obtained with the help of Python and thus justified the proposed system's performances while training, validation, and final stage testing.

3.3.1 Data-Flow Modeling

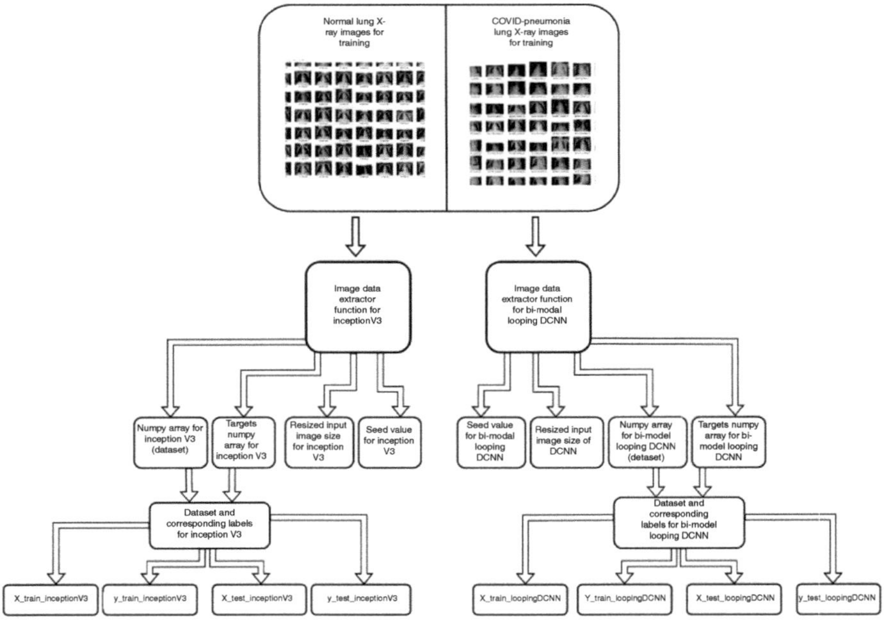

FIGURE 3.2 The entire data-flow modelling of the proposed system.

In Figure 3.2 the entire dataset modeling is demonstrated using block diagrams and thus justifies how we have performed the data engineering and preprocessing. The folder containing all the required images is passed as a parameter to our custom function that can process this folder's contents, the images, and correspondingly convert them into NumPy array to ensure the proper training of the model. We have created two functions: one for obtaining the NumPy array for the InceptionV3 network and the other for the Bi-Modal Looping DCNN. The total number of images that were present in the training folder was around 8,000, belonging to both classes. Implementation of the function that we have coined as the "Image Data Extractor Function" is also provided below. The entire implementation of the function is done in Python along with the help of some core python libraries like OpenCV-Python, Pillow, Numpy, Matplotlib, Tensorflow, etc. The image resizing is also ensured by the designed function and also the creation of the NumPy arrays of the corresponding training, validation, and final testing datasets. The function also returns the value of the resizing size of each image along with a generation seed for the former. OpenCV is mainly used to read the images in RGB format and thereafter the images are resized to the desired dimensions. Pillow is used to handling the resizing of the images to the required dimension of 300×300×3 and thus once resizing is done, the images are then appended in a list along with their corresponding labels as the target classes, "Normal Lungs" and "COVID-Pneumonia Lungs." Numpy is used to convert the images read by OpenCV into their corresponding training tensors to ensure that the designed system can handle the input while training at the next stage. This image data extractor function is designed in such a way that the entire function can be used for creating image NumPy arrays or tensors for the different datasets as well. In the coming chapters, we will see how we have utilized this particular code and how Python allows us to perform object-oriented programming.

3.3.2 Parameters of the Image Data Extractor Function

The image data extractor function requires six different unique parameters to work, which are as follows:

a. folderPath: This parameter is the link to the path that contains the images directory.
b. random_seed: This parameter justifies the seed for creating the image NumPy array.
c. os_env_backend: This parameter justifies which backend must be used for the proper working of the OS library.
d. resize_size: This parameter controls the resizing value of the images, like resize to [500×500×3] from [1024×1024×3].
e. extension_name: This parameter is used to mention the extension of images that we are dealing with.
f. image_format: This parameter justifies the pillow library to properly convert the images to NumPy array and hence controls the entire image data preprocessing technique.

3.3.3 Implementation of the Image Data Extractor Function in Python

Let us see how we can implement the Image Data Extractor Function for converting all the required images and labels into their corresponding NumPy arrays.

```
"def IMAGE_DATA_EXTRACTOR (folderPath="", random_seed=
1010, os_env_backend="", os_backend="", resize_size=0,
extension_name="", image_format=""):"

      "SEED = random_seed"
      "FP = folderPath"
      "OS_BACKEND = os_backend"
      "OS_ENV_BACKEND = os_env_backend"
      "RSIZE = resize_size"
      "EXTENSION = extension_name"
      "FORMAT = image_format"
```

```
"import numpy as np"
"np.random.seed(SEED)"

"import matplotlib.pyplot as plt"
"import os"
"import cv2"
"from PIL import Image"
"import keras"

"os.environ[OS_ENV_BACKEND] = OS_BACKEND "
    "image_directory_2 = FP+"/""
    "SIZE = RSIZE"
"dataset = []"
"label = []"

    #Iterate through all images in normal lungs x-ray
folder, resize to 300x300x3
    #Then save into the same numpy array 'dataset' but
with label 0

"normalImages = os.listdir(image_directory_2 + 'NORMAL/')
for i, image_name in enumerate(normalImages) :"

"if (image_name.split('.')[1] == EXTENSION):"
"image = cv2.imread(image_directory_2 + 'NORMAL/' +
image_name)"
"image = Image.fromarray(image, FORMAT)"
"image = image.resize((SIZE, SIZE))"
"dataset.append(np.array(image))"
"label.append(0)"

    #Iterate through all images in COVID-19 Pneumonia
lungs x-ray folder, resize to 300x300x3
    #Then save into the same numpy array 'dataset' but
with label 1

"covidPneumoniaImages = os.listdir(image_directory_2 +
'PNEUMONIA/')"
"for i, image_name in enumerate(covidPneumoniaImages):"
"if (image_name.split('.')[1] == EXTENSION):"
    "image = cv2.imread(image_directory_2 + 'PNEUMONIA/
' + image_name)"
"image = Image.fromarray(image, FORMAT)"
"image = image.resize((SIZE, SIZE))"
"dataset.append(np.array(image))"
"label.append(1)"

"return dataset, label, SEED, RSIZE"

"if __name__ == "__main__":"

    # Calling the function
    # Links to the folder containing Parasitized and
Uninfected Folders
```

```
"FPath = """
    "IMAGE_DATA, IMAGE_LABELS, SEED, SIZE = IMAGE_DATA_
EXTRACTOR (folderPath=FPath,
random_seed=1010,
os_env_backend='KERAS_BACKEND',
os_backend='tensorflow',
resize_size=300,
extension_name='jpeg',
image_format='RGB')"
```

Thus, the above code illustrates how we have implemented the "Image Data Extractor Function". The function that we have designed is capable of handling any image resizing and corresponding NumPy array conversion. The function is created in such a way that any user can use it just bypassing the link to the folder containing the respective images to work with. In our scenario we are going to deal with normal lung X-ray images and COVID-19 pneumonia lung X-ray images. All the images were kept in a single folder named "training folder," inside which we have the respective folder for each class of images.

In the training folder, we have created two sub-folders named the "Normal Lung X-ray" and "Pneumonia Lung X-ray," which our designed function catches and thereafter performs the required image processing tasks and resizing. This function ensures that the entire dataset that we are going to work with for the neural network training is in the correct format. The Image Data Extractor Function requires a total of seven parameters, out of which the most important parameters are the "folderPath," "random_seed," "resize_size," and "image format."

- "folderPath" is the parameter that captures the link of the folder that contains the respective class folders with corresponding class images. This parameter is the main parameter of the Image Data Extractor Function as it will guide the function to the respective folder for performing image processing and other required tasks. It is a string value.
- "random seed" is the parameter that controls the seed value with which the resulting NumPy array of the images is generated. If we keep the value constant during the execution of the code, the image NumPy array that will be created would also remain constant, thus ensuring the same generation of the resulting NumPy array that we will be using for the training of both the neural networks, the Inception V3 and the Bi-Modal Looping DCNN. The random seed is an integer value between 0 and +infinity.
- "resize size" is the parameter that we have used in the image data extractor function to perform user-defined image resizing. All the images that are present under the "folderPath" are hence resized to a constant value that we have provided during the execution of the designed function. This parameter is an integer as well and, generally, we keep the value to a certain limit. If we tend to resize the images to a very high value, then the time for training the system would increase exponentially. For our work, we have kept the value to 300, to ensure that all the images are resized to 300×300×3 from 1024×1024×3.

- "image format" ensures that all the images are resized and kept in the "RGB" spectrum and thus helps us to perform efficient image processing and resizing via pillow library. This parameter must not be changed during individual applications. Changing this parameter to any other value will result in exceptions that can hinder the entire data preprocessing stage.

3.4 METHODOLOGY

3.4.1 The Inception V3 Architecture and the Bi-Modal Looping DCNN Architecture

When CNNs are trained properly on high-quality data of images, the accuracy of the respective task increases and sometimes even overshoots the current state-of-the-art algorithms. Google gave the idea about a CNN that can go very deep (150+ layers), and thus not only the depth of the layers is increased, but also the architecture was designed in such a way that the parameters formed in each layer are decreased than the previous one, thereby resulting in a total reduction of layer parameters. When we tend to increase the depth of a neural network, the main problem that can be encountered is the problem of getting overfitted. But, Google's Inception V3 Network has got some special components in the architecture that help the overall network in reducing the parameters obtained in each layer. The name "Inception" was derived based on the movie *Inception* by Leonardo DiCaprio, depicting how a person can get multiple linked dreams that affect the net result in a very peculiar way. Inception V3 was first proposed as GoogLeNet and with further modifications and improvisations, version 3 was released and open-sourced for transfer learning purposes. First, the colored image of dimension 299×299×3 was passed to the network's input layer. The image size is then reduced sequentially, first, convolutional layer with features of 32, size of 3×3, and stride of 2×2; second, convolutional layer with features of 32, size of 3×3, and stride of 1×1; third, convolutional layer with features of 64, size of 3×3, and stride of 1×1. Thus, the image dimensions are getting reduced, but the feature maps are increased during this convolutional procedure. Max pooling layers are also used quite often in the network, thus reducing the dimensions and increasing the feature maps a bit. The entire Inception V3 Architecture consists of convolutional layers and max pooling layers operating upon the provided image in different stages. Inception V3 network has mainly five important parameter tuning and reducing components. Inception Block A, Inception Block B, and Inception Block C are the three main blocks for increasing the feature vector in such a way that the overall depth of the network is increased. Reduction Block A and Reduction Block B are the two components of Inception V3 that are responsible for the reduction of parameters of the supplied images. The network is a bit special when observed from the endpoint. The network is comprised of two different dense network classifiers: the Auxiliary Classifier and the Main Classifier. The Auxiliary Classifier acts as the first dream as depicted in the aforementioned movie, the outputs of which indirectly affect the outputs of the main classifier. Google proposed that the number of auxiliary classifiers can be increased depending on the problem and also the resources must be upgraded accordingly. Let us see the detailed overview of this Inception V3 CNN.

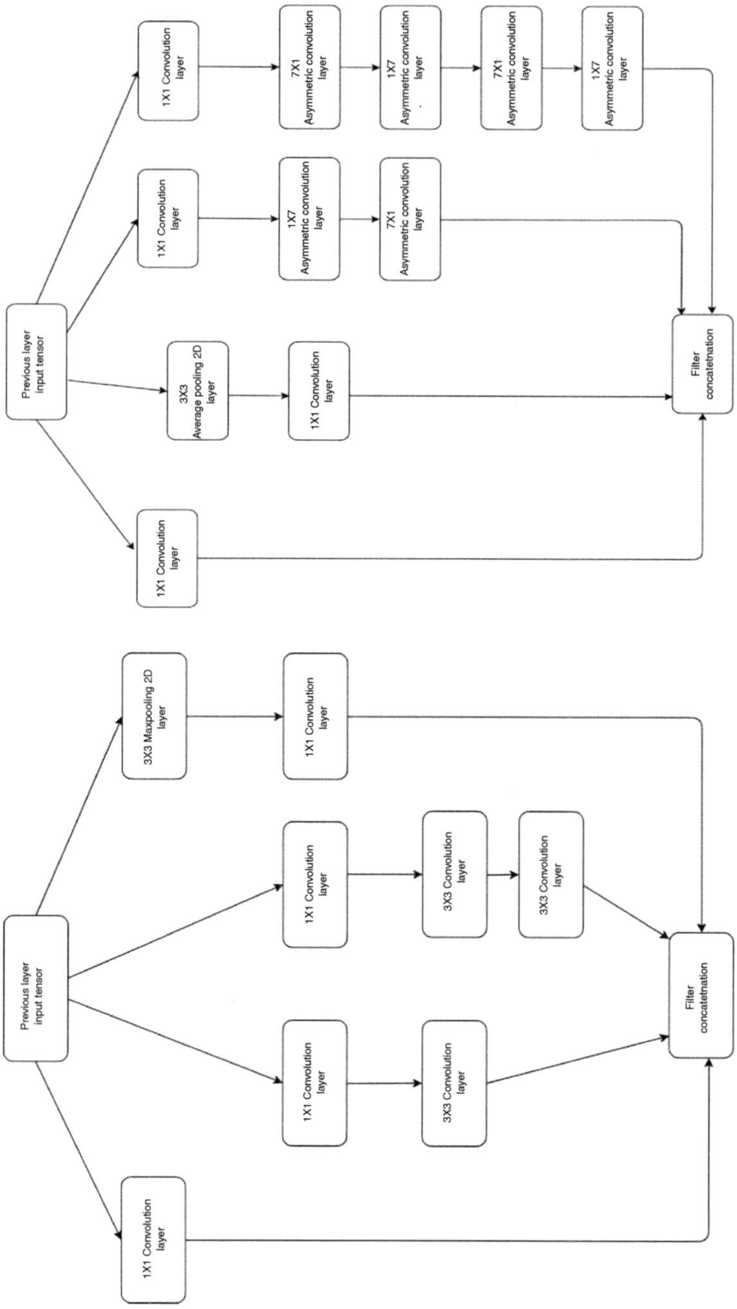

FIGURE 3.3 The Inception Block A (left) and the Inception Block B (right).

In Figure 3.3, Inception Block A and Inception Block B are shown in detail. Both the blocks accept inputs from the previous layers as four-dimensional tensors like [25000,299,299,3], where 25000 is the batch size of images and 299,299,3 depicts the image size. The concept of using multiple-sized convolutional kernels simultaneously is being utilized in these two blocks. The Inception Block A consists of only max pooling and convolutional layers, applied upon the image simultaneously, at different stages. First, 1×1 convolution is used in a branched manner upon the same previous input. The 1×1 convolution acts as a parameter reducer and thus the entire image dimensions are reduced. The block also uses a 3×3 max pooling layer that is capable of further reducing the size and also capturing certain dominant features of the image. Convolutional layers are also used in this block but with a fixed kernel size of 3×3 for increasing the feature vector and reducing the dimensions as well. Thus, all the outputs of the corresponding convolutional layers and max pooling layers are concatenated at the last, yielding another four-dimensional tensor, like [25000, 147,147,64], where 147×147 is the final reduced size of the tensor with corresponding 64 convolutional feature maps capturing different important features. The Inception Block B is mainly there for reducing the parameters again. This block uses the concept of asymmetric convolutions applied simultaneously on the input to the block. The three asymmetric convolutions are divided into two groups for two paths: one followed by 1×7 and 7×1 asymmetric convolutions and the other consisting of a repeated block of these 1×7 and 7×1 asymmetric convolutions that is capable of reducing the parameters to a great extent. This particular block uses this concept of factoring convolutions into multiple asymmetric convolutions. In the earlier versions of Inception, this modification was not introduced and hence we can consider this as an additional improvisation to the existing architecture. This layer also takes a four-dimensional tensor as input and finally after performing the entire procedural operations, the outputs of the respective blocks are once again concatenated. Inception Block C is provided to the architecture just as a modification to the previous reduction component, the asymmetrical convolutions. In this particular block, the layers are mainly convolutional and max pooling, the convolutional layers are there to again reduce the dimensions and thereafter increase the overall final features of the tensor provided as input to the block. This particular block acts as a hybrid of Block A and Block B as depicted in mainly focusing on the asymmetrical convolutional layers. In the block, the 3×3 convolutions are replaced by a block of 1×3 and 3×1 convolutions that try to reduce the overall percentage of parameters in the block. Figure 3.4 presents Inception Block C and how the asymmetrical convolutions happen simultaneously.

In Inception V3 Network, the dimension reduction of the images depends on the reduction blocks of the network. In the network, two reduction blocks, Reduction Block A and Reduction Block B as depicted in Figure 3.5, are there for the main purpose of reducing the dimensions of the increased featured output of the internal blocks. Both the reduction blocks are applied in different stages in the network after the application of the corresponding inception blocks. Reduction Block A utilizes the same power of convolutional layers along with 3×3 max pooling layers that capture further features with increased feature maps and reduced tensor dimensions. The reduction blocks also use the same concepts as the inception blocks, the concept of reducing parameters of the layers such that the network can be made deeper and also wider

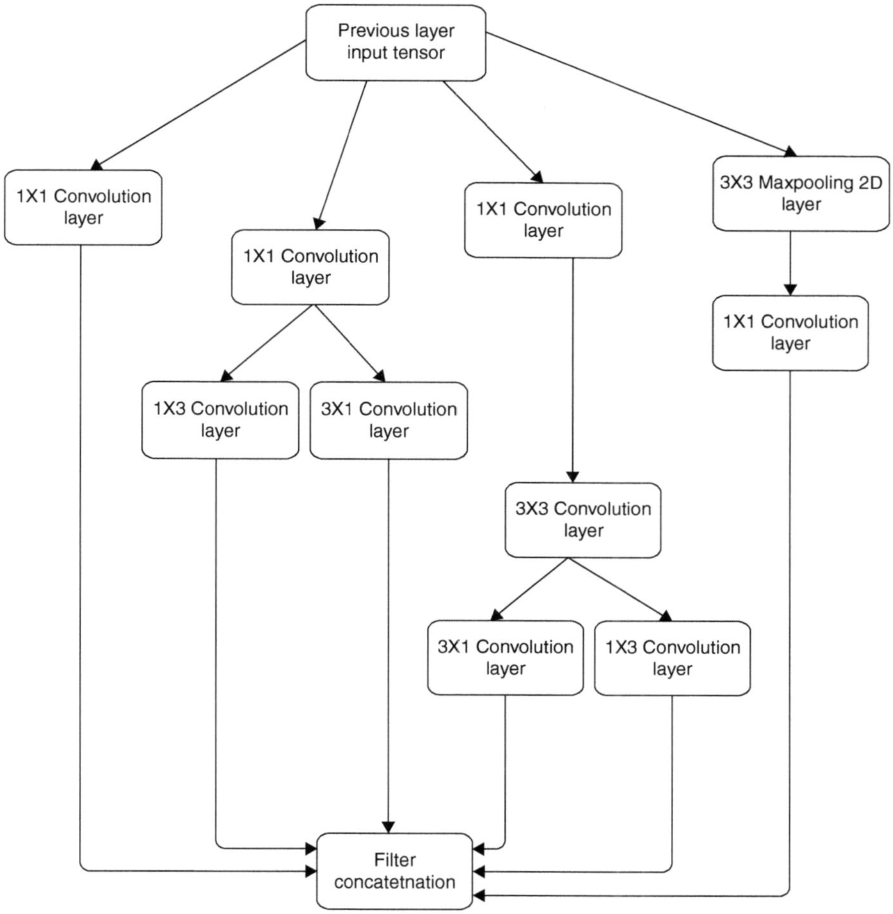

FIGURE 3.4 The Inception Block C.

and the usage of multiple sized convolutional kernels for determining further details. Reduction Block B uses the same concept of asymmetrical convolutions and thus this asymmetrical convolution also tries to reduce the total number of parameters obtained at the ultimate concatenation of layer outputs. Reduction Block B uses the same convolutional layers with max pooling applied at certain intervals, but with a modification of 1×7 and 7×1 asymmetrical convolution blocks repeated for around one time after performing a 1×1 convolution. Thus, both Reduction Block A and Reduction Block B act simultaneously upon the inputs provided to their corresponding blocks. The outputs of the reduction blocks are also concatenated and henceforth passed to the later layers. Thus, with these blocks ready, we can now design the entire Inception V3 architecture, and hence in the structure, the five components can now be placed in their respective manners and thus the entire Inception V3 can be formed. Figure 3.6 depicts how one can design the entire Inception V3 architecture for their respective problem-solving experiments and also how to utilize the aforementioned blocks for

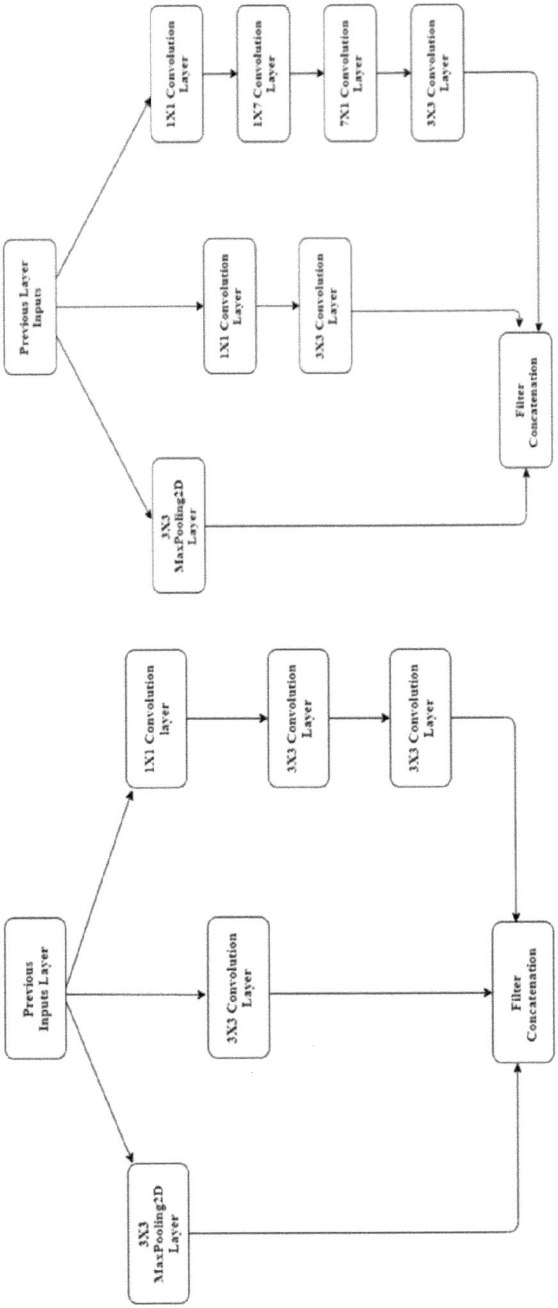

FIGURE 3.5 The Inception V3 Reduction Block A (left) and the Inception V3 Reduction Block B (right).

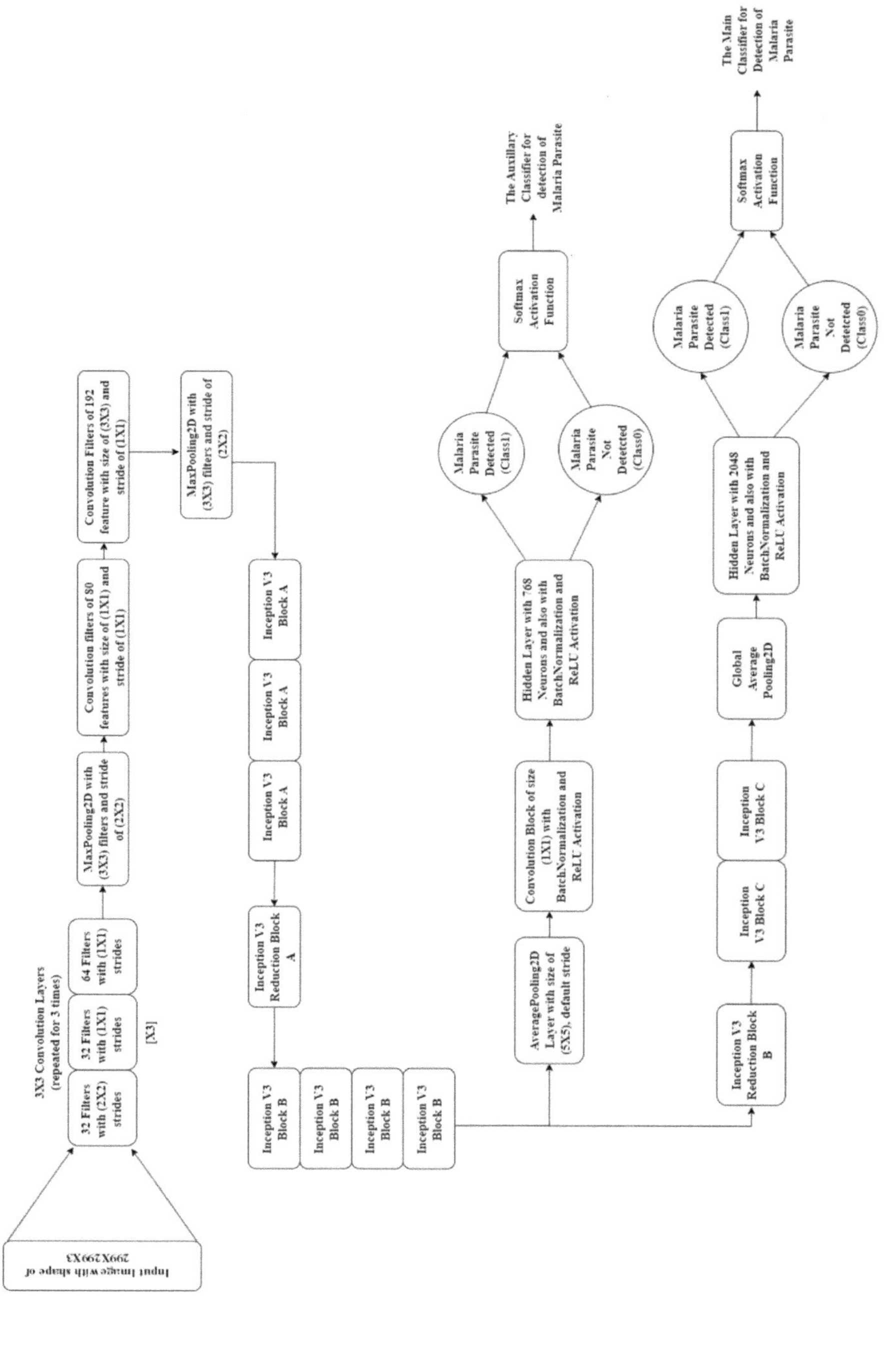

FIGURE 3.6 The Inception V3 architecture in detail.

overall parameter reduction and feature map extension such that the network is capable of performing the task of "Going Deeper with Convolutions."

The entire Inception V3 architecture is depicted in Figure 3.6 with all the incorporation of the blocks, the three inception blocks, and the two reduction blocks. The architecture mainly focuses on the reduction of the layer parameters along with simultaneously increasing the feature maps by utilizing the reduction blocks. Inception V3 requires inputs to be passed in the dimension 299×299×3. This input is passed on to the 3×3 convolutional layer blocks that encompass the reduction of dimension from 299×299×3 to 147×147×64, with 64 representing the convolutional feature maps and the dimension is getting reduced by 50%. The outputs of the convolutional blocks are then passed to the max pooling two-dimensional (2D) layer for further reduction of parameters from 147×147×64 to 78×78×64 for going much deeper into convolutions. The output of the max pooling 2D layer is then passed to the next convolutional blocks that reduce the dimensions further and hence the entire output of the system is provided to the Inception Block A which are getting repeated four times and followed with the implementation of the Reduction Block A, which thereafter increases the feature maps, as well as the dimensionality reduction, is achieved parallelly. After the data is passed and processed by Inception Block A and Reduction Block A, the outputs are then passed to Inception Block B, which is again getting repeated around four times, ensuring further reduction of parameters and depth of the network as well. This reduction of parameters happens due to the presence of asymmetrical convolutions applied to the data. This reduction of parameters is mainly handled by Inception Block B and Reduction Block A. The outputs of the Inception Block B are then separately passed to the auxiliary path which then follows the auxiliary classifier, and the other is passed to the Reduction Block B which again reduces the parameters and ensures that greater depth can be achieved by the network. The Reduction Block B acts just like the Inception Block B, utilizing the same 1×7 and 7×1 asymmetrical convolutions for reduction of dimensions and layer parameters. This reduction of parameters is ensured by Reduction Block B so as to make the data suitable enough for Inception Block C. Inception Block C acts as an ultimate component for reducing the parameters of the overall network and also ensures that the aforementioned system can be repeated many more times to increase the depth further and also the reduction of parameters of the layers.

Inception Block C utilizes the concept of factorization into asymmetric convolutions from 3×3 to two layers having 1×3 and 3×1 asymmetrical convolutions, thus decreasing the percentage of parameters. Thus, the outputs of the Inception Block C are then passed to the final classifier for the final prediction. Inception V3 network can be considered as a way of getting very deep with convolution operations so that one can understand the different hidden features present in the provided image. How Inception V3 network works is a bit advanced but yet effective as previously when people designed very deep neural networks the main problems that appear is the problem of overfitting and decrease in the overall performance of the network during the validation phase.

3.4.2 Implementation of Inception V3 Using Python and Transfer Learning

In this section, we will be looking at the Python code for the implantation of Inception V3 network via the method of transfer learning. Python provides us with the simplicity of using the aforementioned state-of-the-art image detection algorithm with great ease. For the usage, we have used the Tensorflow applications module which is a part of Keras but using the Tensorflow backend. Along with Inception V3, we can even use the pre-trained model that is being trained upon millions of images during the ImageNet competition, or we can also perform training from scratch upon the required custom dataset.

```
"import tensorflow.keras as keras"
"from tensorflow.keras.applications.inception_v3 import
InceptionV3"
"from tensorflow.keras.layers import Dense, Flatten,
LeakyReLU, BatchNormalization, Dropout"

# load model without classifier layers

"model_inception = InceptionV3(include_top=False, input_
shape=(SIZE, SIZE, 3))"

# add new classifier layers

"flat1 = Flatten()(model_inception.layers[-1].output)"
"output_inception = Dense(2, activation='softmax')(flat1)"

# we can add more dense layers as well for increasing the
total parameters of the system
# define new model

"ModelInceptionV3 = Model(inputs=model_inception.inputs,
outputs=output_inception)"

# summarize

"ModelInceptionV3.summary()"
```

Thus, with the above code in hand we can now train the Inception V3 model upon our custom dataset, i.e., the detection of normal lungs X-ray images and COVID-19 pneumonia lungs X-ray images. Thus, our custom Inception V3 has been created and we can now perform the compilation of the entire model and hence continue the training thereafter. We have used the adaptive moments optimization technique for the compilation of the model.

Let us take a look at the compilation of the created Inception V3 model.

```
"ModelInceptionV3.compile(optimizer=tf.keras.optimizers.
Adam(learning_rate=0.001,
beta_1=0.85,
beta_2=0.9,
epsilon=1.15e-08,
decay=1.15e-08),
loss=tf.keras.losses.SparseCategoricalCrossentropy(from_
logits=False),
metrics=['accuracy', 'mae'])"
```

We have provided some arguments to the Adam Optimizer, like the learning rate, beta_1 and beta_2 values, epsilon, and Decay for the better performance of the model and these values are empirical and can be treated as hyperparameters of the system. We have also provided a deeper intuition behind the mathematics that is used in the functioning of the Adam Optimizer.

Finally, for the training of the model, we have used the standard way of training. The model that we have created inherits a function named the fit function. Using this fit function, we have performed the entire training of the Inception V3 model along with parallel training of the custom-designed Bi-Modal Looping DCNN model. We will also see how to implement the Bi-Modal Looping DCNN network that would act as a support to our Inception V3 network.

Let us see how to perform the final training of the Inception V3 network again using Python.

```
#Fitting the model that we have created
"history2 = ModelInceptionV3.fit (x = X_train,
                                   y = y_train,
batch_size = 32,
verbose = 1,
epochs = 100,
validation_data = (X_validation, y_validation),
shuffle=True)"
```

Thus, the history2 parameter stores all the values of the performance metrics like training_accuracy, validation_accuracy, training_loss, and validation_loss. Thus, the training of the Inception V3 is completed and then we can start the designing of the Bi-Modal Looping DCNN that would work on the same images but with two convolutional paths.

The Bi-Modal Looping DCNN uses two convolutional paths for capturing the corresponding features of the images. The name "Bi-Modal" suggests that the network would work on two images of the same categories simultaneously ensuring better performance during training. Residual networks, a way proposed by Kaiming He, played a major role in learning image features just by going deeper with convolutions but with a slight modification in the architecture, the skip connection, also known as the Identity Block. The Bi-Modal Looping DCNN uses the principle of this residual network but in a parallel convolutional channeled way. The Bi-Modal Looping DCNN has two convolutional paths, both of which use the same dimension of convolution operation in their respective channels. Many skip connections are also provided in both the paths so as to ensure proper functionality of the backpropagation and also to reduce the chance of vanishing and exploding gradients problems. We can conclude that the Bi-Modal Looping DCNN works just according to how residual networks work and thus we are able to perform better detection of COVID-pneumonia X-ray images and normal lung X-ray images.

The total number of parameters that the Bi-Modal Looping DCNN exhibits is greater than 3M and thus, along with Inception V3 as another component, the total parameters of the system were found to be more than 25M. With such a great number of parameters, we have to ensure that the number of images that we are working on also increases in time, thus ensuring better training and optimization.

Let us see how we have implemented the Bi-Modal Looping DCNN for the detection of COVID-19 pneumonia using Python and Tensorflow.

```
"import tensorflow.keras as keras"
"import tesnorflow as tf"

"inputs = keras.Input(shape=(SIZE, SIZE, 3), name="img1")"
"inputs2 = keras.Input(shape=(SIZE, SIZE, 3), name=
"img2")"

"x =keras.layers.Conv2D(32, 3, activation="relu")(inputs)"
"x = keras.layers.Conv2D(64, 3, activation="relu")(x)"
"block_1_output = keras.layers.MaxPooling2D(2)(x)"
"x = keras.layers.Conv2D(64, 3, activation="relu",
padding="same")(block_1_output)"
"x = keras.layers.Conv2D(64, 3, activation="relu",
padding="same")(x)"
"block_2_output = keras.layers.add([x, block_1_output])"
"x = keras.layers.Conv2D(64, 3, activation="relu",
padding="same")(block_2_output)"
"x = keras.layers.Conv2D(64, 3, activation="relu",
padding="same")(x)"
"block_3_output = keras.layers.add([x, block_2_output])"
"x = keras.layers.Conv2D(64, 3, activation="relu",
padding="same")(block_3_output)"
"x = keras.layers.Conv2D(64, 3, activation="relu",
padding="same")(x)"
"block_4_output = keras.layers.add([x, block_3_output])"
"x = keras.layers.Conv2D(64, 3, activation="relu",
padding="same")(block_4_output)"
"x = keras.layers.Conv2D(64, 3, activation="relu",
padding="same")(x)"
"block_5_output = keras.layers.add([x, block_4_output])"
"x = keras.layers.Conv2D(64, 3, activation="relu",
padding="same")(block_5_output)"
"x = keras.layers.Conv2D(64, 3, activation="relu",
padding="same")(x)"
"block_6_output = keras.layers.add([x, block_5_output])"
"x = keras.layers.Conv2D(64, 3, activation="relu",
padding="same")(block_2_output)"
"x = keras.layers.Conv2D(64, 3, activation="relu",
padding="same")(x)"
"block_7_output = keras.layers.add([x, block_6_output])"
"x = keras.layers.Conv2D(64, 3, activation="relu",
padding="same")(block_1_output)"
"x = keras.layers.Conv2D(64, 3, activation="relu",
padding="same")(x)"
"block_8_output = keras.layers.add([x, block_7_output])"
"x=keras.layers.Conv2D(64,3,activation="relu")(block_8_
output)"
"x = keras.layers.GlobalAveragePooling2D()(x)"
"x = keras.layers.Dense(256, activation="relu")(x)"
"x1 = keras.layers.Dropout(0.5)(x)"
"x=keras.layers.Conv2D(64, 3, activation="relu")(inputs2)"
"x = keras.layers.Conv2D(64, 3, activation="relu")(x)"
```

```
"block_1_output = keras.layers.MaxPooling2D(2)(x)"
"x = keras.layers.Conv2D(64, 3, activation="relu",
padding="same")(block_1_output)"
"x = keras.layers.Conv2D(64, 3, activation="relu",
padding="same")(x)"
"block_2_output = keras.layers.add([x, block_1_output])"
"x = keras.layers.Conv2D(64, 3, activation="relu",
padding="same")(block_2_output)"
"x = keras.layers.Conv2D(64, 3, activation="relu",
padding="same")(x)"
"block_3_output = keras.layers.add([x, block_2_output])"
"x = keras.layers.Conv2D(64, 3, activation="relu",
padding="same")(block_3_output)"
"x = keras.layers.Conv2D(64, 3, activation="relu",
padding="same")(x)"
"block_4_output = keras.layers.add([x, block_3_output])"
"x = keras.layers.Conv2D(64, 3, activation="relu",
padding="same")(block_3_output)"
"x = keras.layers.Conv2D(64, 3, activation="relu",
padding="same")(x)"
"block_5_output = keras.layers.add([x, block_4_output])"
"x = keras.layers.Conv2D(64, 3, activation="relu",
padding="same")(block_3_output)"
"x = keras.layers.Conv2D(64, 3, activation="relu",
padding="same")(x)"
"block_6_output = keras.layers.add([x, block_5_output])"
"x = keras.layers.Conv2D(64, 3, activation="relu",
padding="same")(block_2_output)"
"x = keras.layers.Conv2D(64, 3, activation="relu",
padding="same")(x)"
"block_7_output = keras.layers.add([x, block_6_output])"
"x = keras.layers.Conv2D(64, 3, activation="relu",
padding="same")(block_1_output)"
"x = keras.layers.Conv2D(64, 3, activation="relu",
padding="same")(x)"
"block_8_output = keras.layers.add([x, block_7_output])"
"x=keras.layers.Conv2D(64,3,activation="relu")(block_8_output)"
"x = keras.layers.GlobalAveragePooling2D()(x)"
"x = keras.layers.Dense(256, activation="relu")(x)"
"x2 = keras.layers.Dropout(0.5)(x)"
"concat1 = keras.layers.concatenate([x1, x2])"
"x = keras.layers.Dense(512, activation="relu")(concat1)"
"x = keras.layers.Dropout(0.5)(x)"

"outputs = keras.layers.Dense(2, activation='softmax')(x)"
"model3=keras.Model([inputs,inputs2], outputs, name=
"Looping-DCNN-Chest-Xray")"
"model3.summary()"

"model3.compile(optimizer=keras.optimizers.Adam(learning_
rate=0.001,

beta_1=0.85,
```

```
beta_2=0.9,
epsilon=1.15e-08,
decay=1.15e-08),
loss= tf.keras.losses.SparseCategoricalCrossentropy(from_
logits=False),
metrics=['accuracy'])"
```

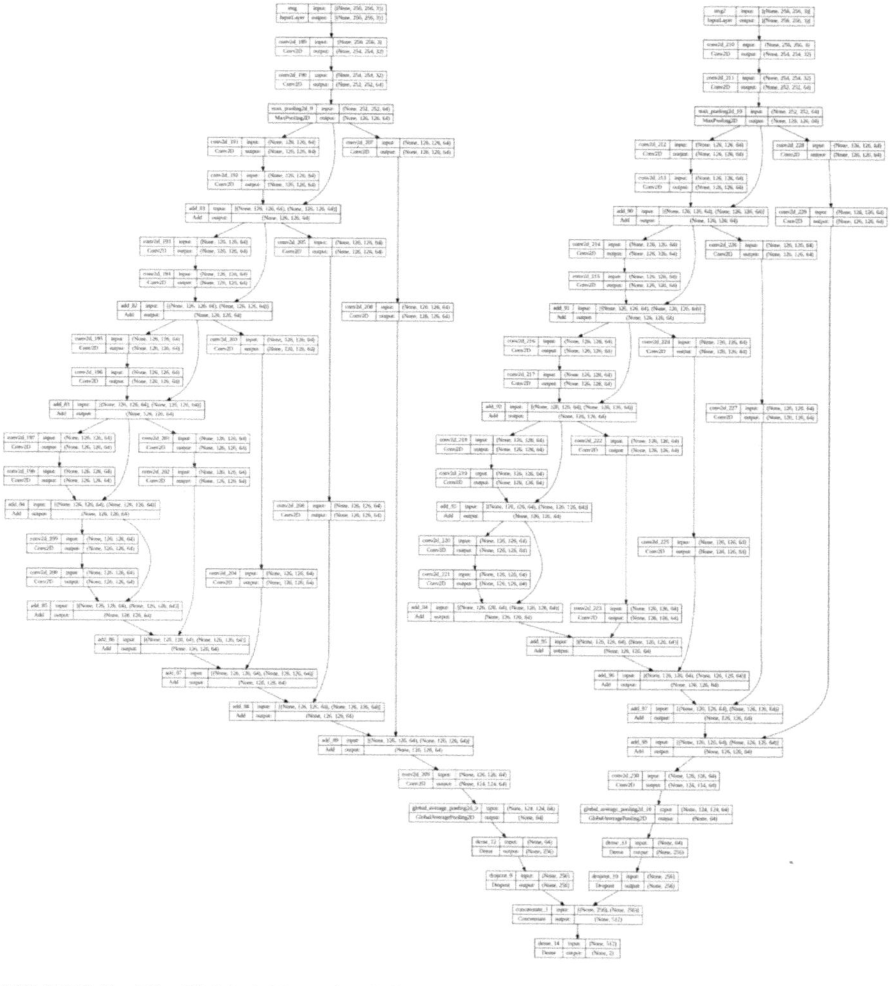

FIGURE 3.7 The Bi-Modal Looping DCNN architecture in detail.

Thus, once the compilation is done successfully, we can perform the training of the model just like we did in the case of Inception V3. We are going to use the fit function as a tool to train this model as well and thus, once the training is done, the Bi-Modal Looping DCNN is ready to perform detection of the supplied images. This prediction that we are performing is done totally by the network via those multiple convolutional paths and thus ensuring better convergence of the gradients during the backpropagation phase. Thus, we can see how we have implemented the entire Bi-Modal Looping DCNN. The diagram that we have created for a better understanding of the designed convolutional network, Figure 3.7, depicts the designed Bi-Modal Looping DCNN that will work in coherence with the Inception V3 network, thus ensuring better-tuned predictions for the supplied inputs. The design of the Bi-Modal Looping DCNN incorporates the principle of residual networks but at a much sophisticated level. Skip connections are added sequentially to ensure better feature capturing during the training and prediction stages. In the next section, we have also provided a block diagram for the working of the entire Bi-Modal Looping DCNN. For better understanding do have a careful look at the block diagram of the aforementioned model. The block diagram depicts how the skip connections are added and thereafter how the entire network is understood at a much deeper level. The block diagrams that we have provided are also acting as a support for a better understanding of the complex model. Let us have a look at the designed network's block diagram which is provided in Figure 3.8.

3.4.3 The Adaptive Moments Optimization Technique (aka Adam Optimizer)

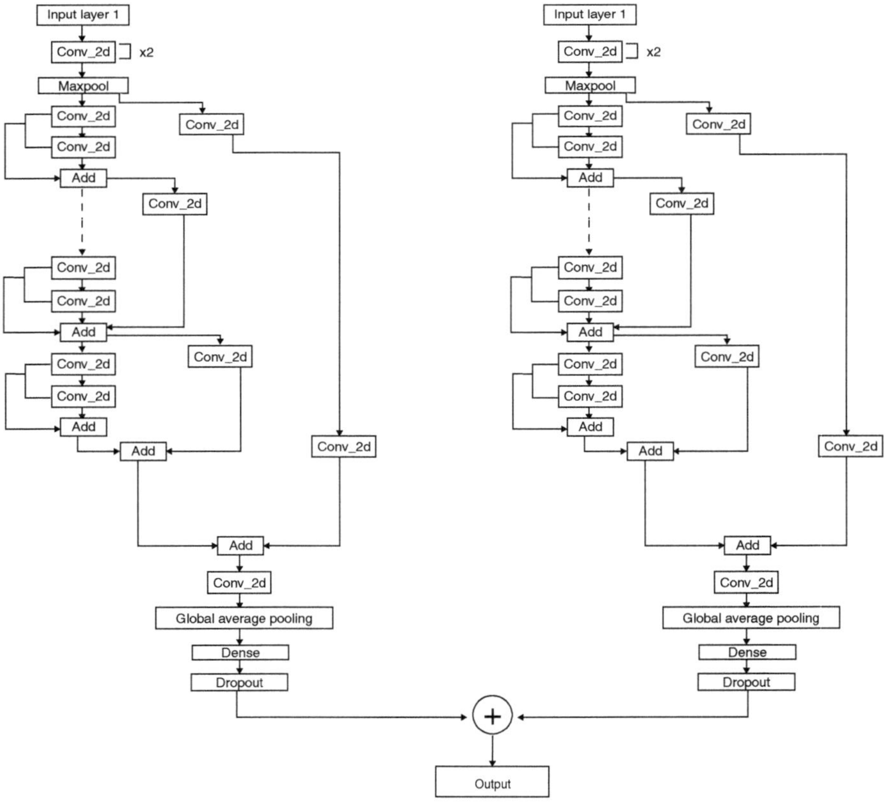

FIGURE 3.8 The rntire block diagram for the custom-designed Bi-Modal Looping DCNN.

The proposed system acts like an Ensemble System during the final stage prediction. Creating ensembles of CNNs solves the problem of misclassification by detecting common features at a much higher level. Our proposed system can not only tackle outliers but also reduce the chances of overfitting up to a great extent. In Section 3.5, we have also provided the performance metrics graphs so as to support our proposals. The graphs were generated using Python and matplotlib and they justify how the neural network performs during the training phase and how the validation accuracy and the corresponding validation loss are measured. But before we can jump to the result analysis portion, we can have a look at the use of adaptive moments optimization technique and the related mathematical formulations. In the next section, we will see how the internal mathematics of the Adam Optimizer is performed.

3.4.3.1 The Adaptive Moments Optimization aka ADAM Optimizer Algorithm

Require: Step size
Require: $\beta_1, \beta_2 \in [0,1)$: Exponential decay rates for the moment estimates
Require: $f(\theta)$: Stochastic objective function with parameters θ
Require: θ_0 : Initial parameter vector
$m_0 \leftarrow 0$ (Initialize 1st moment vector)
$v_0 \leftarrow 0$ (Initialize 2nd moment vector)
$t \leftarrow 0$ (Initialize timestep)
while θ_t not converged
do { $t \leftarrow t+1 g_t \leftarrow \nabla_\theta f_t(\theta_{t-1})$ (Get gradients w.r.t. stochastic objective at time step t)

$m_t \leftarrow \beta_1 \cdot m_{t-1} + (1-\beta_1) \cdot g_t$ (Update biased first moment estimate)
$v_t \leftarrow \beta_2 \cdot v_{t-1} + (1-\beta_2) \cdot g_t^2$ (Update biased second raw moment estimate)
$\hat{m}_t \leftarrow m_t / (1-\beta_1^t)$ (Compute bias-corrected first moment estimate)
$\hat{v}_t \leftarrow v_t / (1-\beta_2^t)$ (Compute bias-corrected second raw moment estimate)
$\theta_t \leftarrow \theta_{t-1} - \alpha \cdot \hat{m}_t / (\sqrt{\hat{v}_t} + \epsilon)$ (Update parameters)
end while

Return θ_t (Resulting parameters)

}

RMSprop and stochastic gradient descent are combined in the ADAM Optimizer. Similar to RMSprop, it scales the learning rate using squared gradients and, like SGD with momentum, it takes advantage of momentum by using the moving average of the gradient rather than the gradient itself. Let's examine its operation in more detail. This optimizer computes individual learning rates for various parameters according to an adaptive learning rate algorithm. Because ADAM employs estimations of the first and second moments of the gradient to change the learning rate for each weight of the neural network, it gets its name from the phrase "adaptable moment estimation."

More formally:

$$m_n = E[X^n]$$

where m = moment and X = random variable.

Any deep neural network's gradients can be thought of as a random variable. The first instant is the actual mean, while the second is the uncluttered variance (in which case the mean is not subtracted when calculating the variance). The ADAM Optimizer uses exponentially weighted moving averages, computed on the gradient evaluated on a contemporary mini-batch, to estimate the moments considerably more precisely. The fundamental formulation that we employed in our suggested work is the same as that presented in ADAM Optimizer's original study. This optimization approach is used in the very first step of our conceptual scheme, Multimodal System, which is the training of our three separate CNNs. The following list contains the ADAM basic formulas.

$$m_t = \beta_1 m_{t-1} + (1-\beta_1) g_t \, V_t = \beta_2 V_{t-1} + (1-\Delta_2) g_t^2$$

where g is the gradient on the current mini-batch, m and v are moving averages, and β_1 and β_2 are newly introduced hyperparameters of the algorithm.

A. Moving Averages of Gradient and Squared Gradient

Beta 1 and Beta 2 have excellent default values of 0.9 and 0.999. At the beginning of the iteration, moving average vectors are initialized with zeros. Let's look at the expected values of our moving averages to determine how these values correspond to the current situation. Since m and v are estimates of the first and second moments, we want to have the following property:

$$E[m_t] = E[g_t] \, E[v_t] = E[g_t^2]$$

In our situation, the parameter is also the expected value, which is surprising because the expected values of the estimators should match the parameter we're trying to estimate. These qualities would indicate the existence of unbiased estimators if they were true. We'll see in a moment that these do not apply to our moving averages. The estimators are skewed toward zero because we start averages with zeros. We also made an analytical and condensed attempt to demonstrate the entirety of the aforementioned concept. The following is the primary extension of the entire ADAM concept.

$$\begin{aligned} m_0 &= 0 m_1 = \beta_1 m_0 + (1-\beta_1) g_1 \\ &= (1-\beta_1) g_1 \, m_2 = \beta_1 m_1 + (1-\beta_1) g_2 \\ &= \beta_1 (1-\beta_1) g_1 + (1-\beta_1) g_2 \, m_3 = \beta_1 m_2 + (1-\beta_1) g_3 \\ &= \beta_1^2 (1-\beta_1) g_1 + \beta_1 (1-\beta_1) g_2 + (1-\beta_1) g_3 \end{aligned}$$

The more "far" we spread the value of m, the less the early values of gradients contribute to the overall value because they are multiplied by a less and smaller amount of beta. In order to account for this pattern, we can update the formula for our moving average as shown below. Doing so will enable us to create the ADAM Optimizer for our ensemble CNN system.

$$m_t = (1-\beta_1)\sum_{i=0}^{t}\beta_1^{t-i} g_i$$

Let's take a look at the expected value of *m*, to see how it relates to the true first moment, so we can correct for the discrepancy of the two:

$$E[m_t] = E\left[(1-\beta_1)\sum_{i=1}^{t}\beta_1^{t-i} g_i\right] = E[g_i](1-\beta_1)\sum_{i=1}^{t}\beta_1^{t-i} + \zeta = E[g_i](1-\beta_1)+\zeta$$

B. Bias Correction for the First Momentum Estimator

We enlarge *m* in the first row using our new moving average algorithm. Then, using *g*[*t*], we approximate *g*[*i*]. Given that it no longer depends on *I* we can now remove it from the sum. The formula shows the error *C* as a result of the approximation. The formula for the sum of a finite geometric series is all that is used in the final line. The following will be the estimator's final formulas:

$$\hat{m}_t = \frac{m_t}{1-\beta_1} \quad \hat{v}_t = \frac{v_t}{1-\beta_2}$$

The only thing left to do is to use those moving averages to scale the learning rate individually for each parameter.

$$w_t = w_{t-1} - \eta\frac{\hat{m}_t}{\sqrt{\hat{v}_t + \epsilon}}$$

where η (which resembles the letter n) is the step size and *w* are the model weights (it can depend on iteration). The update rule for Adam that we have utilized in our suggested work is complete. When Inception V3 and the Bi-Modal Looping DCNN are being trained, the ADAM Optimizer is crucial. In our proposed ensemble deep learning system, ADAM Optimizer reduces the loss function produced by the associated CNNs.

C. Final Formulation of the ADAM Optimizer

$$\frac{(I_t, \alpha_t, \beta_1, \beta_2, \epsilon)}{m_0 = 0, v_0 = 0}$$

$$m_{t+1} = \beta_1 m_t + (1-\beta_1)\nabla l(\theta_t)$$

$$v_{t+1} = \beta_2 v_t + (1-\beta_2)\nabla l(\theta_t)^2$$

$$b_{t+1} = \frac{\sqrt{1-\beta_2^{t+1}}}{1-\beta_1^{t+1}}$$

$$\theta_{t+1} = \theta_t - \alpha_t \frac{m_{t+1}}{\sqrt{v_{t+1}} + \epsilon} b_{t+1}$$

3.5 RESULT ANALYSIS

The total number of parameters of the Looping DCNN was found to be 590,466 and all of them being trainable. The Looping DCNN was designed using the principle of the same convolutions applied in a nested format to the inner layers. The parameters of the network are reduced accordingly by using convolution operations with the same number of kernels and kernel dimensions, thus allowing us to go deeper yet reducing the parameters. During the training, at certain points, our proposed system tends to lag down a bit while validating, but in due time the training and validation seem to be converging. The principle of convolution is just matrix multiplication and replacing each value of the convolution matrix with the corresponding convoluted values. CNNs are always preferred over any other traditional deep learning or machine learning algorithms as the target can be easily achieved by a simple CNN as well as a complex logical CNN. Thus, while we were training the first component, it became clear to us that the data set is a bit tricky so no naive or simple model can tackle with it. Deep learning always tends to be a bit more abstract as we cannot formulate such big notations in mathematics, which leads to the concepts of Black Boxes solving some certain tasks.

Figure 3.9 shows the performance graphs of the second component that will act like a support to the Inception V3, the Looping DCNN. The performance graphs of this component seem to be quite interesting.

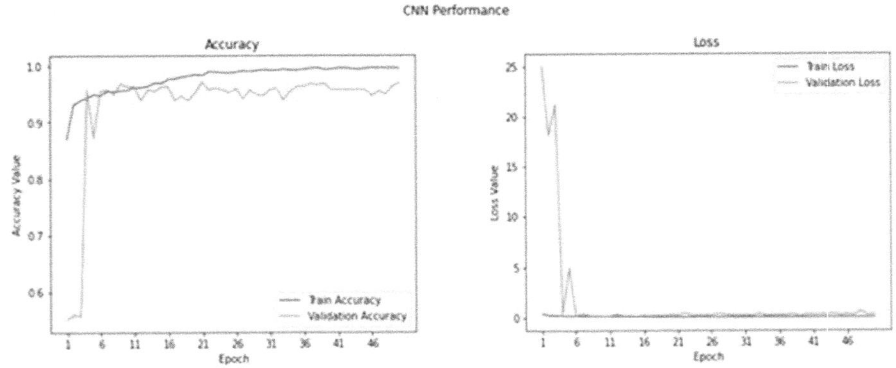

FIGURE 3.9 The performance graphs of the Bimodal Looping DCNN.

From Figure 3.9, it is clear that the training performance was quite impressive. For the training accuracy, the network was able to reach an accuracy of 98.25% with a corresponding loss of 0.0175, while validation accuracy reached a maximum value of 97% with a corresponding validation loss of 0.025. Thus, the performance graphs tell us that notwithstanding being such a deeper and broader network, the Looping DCNN was able to validate on testing samples, and thus the chance of getting overfitting has also been reduced.

The optimizer that we have proposed to use for the Looping DCNN was trained by using the Adam Optimizer with a learning rate of 0.00075, beta_1 and beta_2 being fixed at 0.87 and 0.98, respectively. The optimization algorithm used was Adam as using many other optimization techniques can lead the network to be trained naively. But using the Adam Optimization algorithm, the performance graphs gradually reached the limiting threshold.

Figure 3.10 demonstrates how the performance graphs were for the Inception V3 network. In deep learning, the concept of transfer learning plays a vital role in solving real-world problems. The Inception V3 network proposed by Google was open-sourced in 2014 via Python upon TensorFlow and PyTorch. In this work, we have used the Inception V3 network for the detection of pneumonia from lung X-ray images to identify the presence of COVID-19.

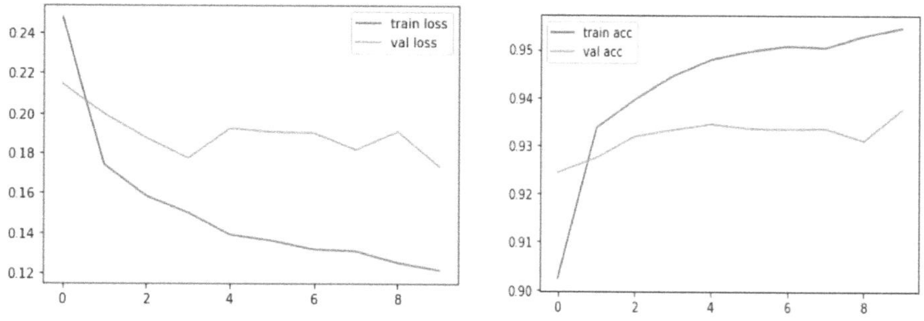

FIGURE 3.10 The performance graphs for the Inception V3 network.

The network architecture of Inception V3 is notably intricate, as previously discussed in detail. Google introduced this network in their paper titled "Going Deeper with Convolutions," which surpassed existing state-of-the-art algorithms. Inception V3 was originally trained on the ImageNet dataset, a substantial collection of high-resolution images spanning approximately 1,000 different categories. The results achieved with Inception V3 were exceptionally robust, leading to its adoption as the new state-of-the-art model. In our work, we employed transfer learning to leverage Inception V3's capabilities. The network comprises approximately 224 layers and operates on the principle of progressively reducing image dimensions while delving deeper with convolutions. During the training of Inception V3, we aimed to minimize the number of epochs required, opting to train the network from scratch. The training process consisted of approximately 35 epochs, employing a conditional decaying learning rate scheduler and early stopping. The results obtained were not only robust but also converged within the desired thresholds for accuracy and loss. Specifically, Inception V3 was trained for approximately 35 epochs, with early stopping applied around the 15th epoch, marking the conclusion of the model's training phase. At this point, the training accuracy reached 98%, and the training loss was 0.054. Meanwhile, the validation accuracy plateaued at approximately

TABLE 3.1
Results obtained during training of the individual convolutional neural networks

Name of the Model	Optimizer Used	Optimizer Configuration	Training Accuracy	Training Loss	Validation Accuracy	Validation Loss
The Bimodal Looping Deep Convolutional Neural Network (DCNN)	Adaptive Moments Optimization (Adam Optimizer)	Learning rate was 0.00075, beta_1 and beta_2 were kept at 0.87 and 0.98, respectively, with a default value of decay and slope	98.25%	0.0175	97%	0.025
The Inception V3	Adam Optimizer	Learning rate was 0.00085, beta_1 and beta_2 was kept at 0.75 and 0.85, respectively, with a default value of epsilon and decay was kept at 1.75e-08	98%	0.054	97.25%	0.0757

97.25%, accompanied by a corresponding validation loss of 0.0757. These results demonstrated the system's capability to detect the presence of COVID-19 features or pneumonia with remarkable accuracy. The training of the ensemble system was conducted on a powerful workstation featuring 64 GB of RAM and an Nvidia Tesla P100 GPU with 16 GB of memory. Due to the extensive resource requirements, further training iterations may not yield significant reductions in time consumption.

The learning rate for Inception V3 training remained fixed at 0.00085, with beta_1 and beta_2 set at 0.75 and 0.85, respectively. Additionally, a decay value of 1.75e-08 and epsilon set to the default value were used in the training process. The final results are provided in Table 3.1 for reference.

3.6 CONCLUSION

From the comprehensive analysis of the COVID X-ray dataset using the ensemble system, it's evident that this dataset can serve as a valuable resource for further research and analysis. The results obtained are quite satisfactory, indicating the potential for meaningful applications.

- To enhance the system's performance, one avenue for improvement is the application of hyperparameter optimization techniques in deep learning. Fine-tuning the model's hyperparameters can lead to even better results, making the system more robust and accurate.
- The incorporation of transfer learning concepts, as demonstrated in this analysis, can significantly outperform other methods for solving domain-specific problems. This approach paves the way for the creation of hyperparameter-optimized systems of neural networks, which can be fine-tuned to excel in specific tasks and domains.

In conclusion, deep learning offers a versatile and powerful toolkit that can be applied in various fields, including the medical field. The analysis of X-ray images, such as those of COVID-19-affected individuals' lungs, using DCNNs, has proven effective in detecting the presence of viral pneumonia. This technology holds great promise for advancing medical research and improving diagnostic capabilities.

REFERENCES

1. Lundervold, A.S. and Lundervold, A., 2019. An overview of deep learning in medical imaging focusing on MRI. *Zeitschrift für Medizinische Physik*, 29(2), pp. 102–127.
2. Greenspan, H., Van Ginneken, B. and Summers, R.M., 2016. Guest editorial deep learning in medical imaging: Overview and future promise of an exciting new technique. *IEEE Transactions on Medical Imaging*, 35(5), pp. 1153–1159.
3. Suzuki, K., 2017. Overview of deep learning in medical imaging. *Radiological Physics and Technology*, 10(3), pp. 257–273.
4. Romanov, A., Bach, M., Yang, S., Franzeck, F.C., Sommer, G., Anastasopoulos, C., Bremerich, J., Stieltjes, B., Weikert, T. and Sauter, A.W., 2021.Automated CT lung density analysis of viral pneumonia and healthy lungs using deep

learning-based segmentation, histograms and HU thresholds. *Diagnostics*, 11(5), p. 738.

5. Khan, A.A., Shafiq, S., Kumar, R., Kumar, J. and Haq, A.U., 2020, December. H3DNN: 3D Deep learning based detection of COVID-19 virus using lungs computed tomography. In *2020 17th International Computer Conference on Wavelet Active Media Technology and Information Processing (ICCWAMTIP)* (pp. 183–186).
6. Al-Waisy, A.S., Al-Fahdawi, S., Mohammed, M.A., Abdulkareem, K.H., Mostafa, S.A., Maashi, M.S., Arif, M. and Garcia-Zapirain, B., 2020. COVID-CheXNet: Hybrid deep learning framework for identifying COVID-19 virus in chest X-rays images.
7. Phillips, N.A., Rajpurkar, P., Sabini, M., Krishnan, R., Zhou, S., Pareek, A., Phu, N.M., Wang, C., Jain, M., Du, N.D. and Truong, S.Q., 2020, November. CheXphoto: 10,000+ Photos and transformations of chest X-rays for benchmarking deep learning robustness.
8. Brunese, L., Mercaldo, F., Reginelli, A. and Santone, A., 2020. Explainable deep learning for pulmonary disease and coronavirus COVID-19 detection from X-rays. *Computer Methods and Programs in Biomedicine*, 196, p. 105608.
9. Yan, C., Yao, J., Li, R., Xu, Z. and Huang, J., 2018, August. Weakly supervised deep learning for thoracic disease classification and localization on chest X-rays. In *Proceedings of the 2018 ACM international conference on bioinformatics, computational biology, and health informatics.*
10. Rajaraman, S., Siegelman, J., Alderson, P.O., Folio, L.S., Folio, L.R. and Antani, S.K., 2020. Iteratively pruned deep learning ensembles for COVID-19 detection in chest X-rays. *IEEE Access*, 8, pp. 115041–115050.
11. Kumar, A., Tripathi, A.R., Satapathy, S.C. and Zhang, Y.D., 2022. SARS-Net: COVID-19 detection from chest X-rays by combining graph convolutional network and convolutional neural network. *Pattern Recognition*, 122, p. 108255.
12. Pham, T.D., 2021. Classification of COVID-19 chest X-rays with deep learning: New models or fine tuning? *Health Information Science and Systems*, 9(1), pp. 1–11.

4 Detection of Pneumonia from a Small-Scale Dataset of X-Ray Images of Lungs by Using a Compound Batch-Normalizing Convolutional Neural Feature Extracting Random Forest Classifier

4.1 INTRODUCTION

In practical deep learning, the amount of data that is required is in terms of thousands and millions. In previously mentioned chapters, the amount of data that we had dealt with was also somewhat near the range of 5000. In this chapter we would delve into the application of deep learning and also transfer learning with the use of around few hundreds of images. Our proposed way can easily solve the challenge of detecting four different categories of lung pneumonia infection. The approach that we have followed is totally dependent of the systems of Convolutional Neural Networks (CNNs), so it is advisable that readers should have a very good knowledge of CNN [1]. In deep learning the main advantage is the automation of feature extraction on domain problems. Deep learning algorithms are quite capable to understand the hidden feature representations, which in turn helps the model learn about different pixel value distributions [2]. The features that are generally present within an image are edges, corners, rounded objects, and so on. But in this particular domain problem, "The Detection of Bacterial and Viral Lung Pneumonia Using Batch-Normalizing Convolutional Neural Feature Extracting Random Forest Classifier (BCNFE-RFC)," we are dealing with X-ray images; so basically detecting only the edges or rounded portions within the images would not at all work; therefore, we are going to experience the entire data in a different format for the system also as mentioned in [3, 4]

DOI: 10.1201/9781003456476-4

and following the basic components of an ensemble system. In this chapter we would also focus on different versions of our proposed domain-specific artificial intelligence (AI) system, including all the different libraries of Python that we have used to implement the entire model. The Python codes are totally defined as functions just so as to ensure the applications of multiprocessing in somewhat future scopes.

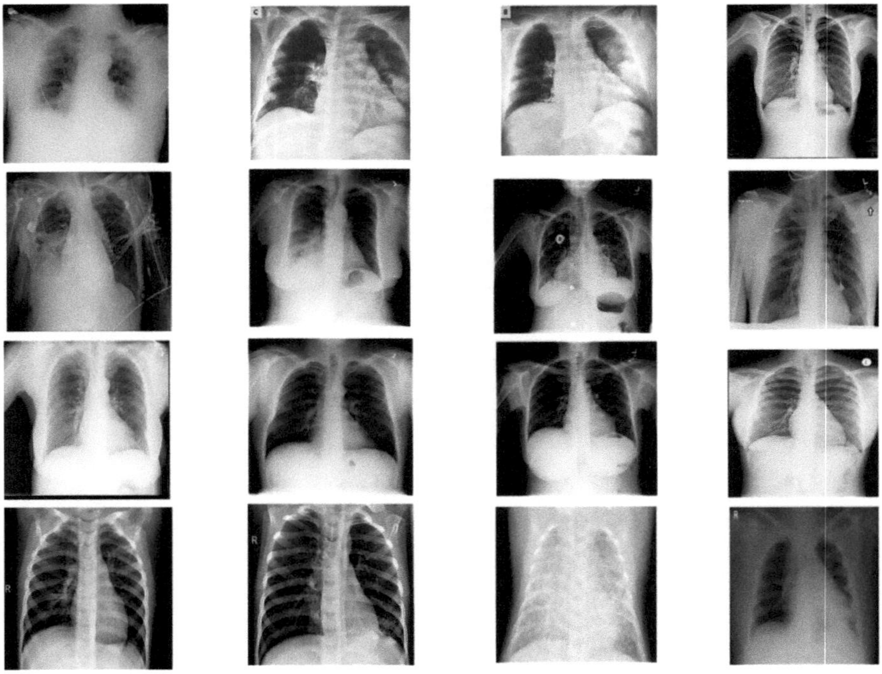

FIGURE 4.1 The X-ray images of four different categories of images we are going to deal with—first row: COVID-19 pneumonia; second row: non-COVID-19 lung pneumonia; third row: the normal lung X-ray; and fourth row: viral pneumonia. All the images were scaled down a bit for better visualizations and preprocessing.

4.2 PNEUMONIA IN LUNGS: A SHORT GUIDE

The prevalence of pneumonia raises serious health concerns. It is an illness that can be fatal and is caused by a number of bacteria and viruses. In situations where it is mistreated or when a timely diagnosis is not made, it may be lethal. When pneumonia is not identified and/or treated in a timely manner, the death rate is significant. Pneumonia comes in a variety of forms, each with its own set of symptoms and warning indications as depicted in Figure 4.1. When a specific lung region swells, pneumonia is identified as the cause. To save the patient's life, it is crucial to detect pneumonia as soon as feasible. It is a fairly widespread illness that is caused by several germs.

4.2.1 Biomedical Agents of Pneumonia

Numerous species, including bacteria, viruses, and fungus, are the causative factors of pneumonia. Bacteria, which can come from the environment, the gastrointestinal (GI) tract, and the respiratory tract, are the most frequent causes of pneumonia. In children virus is the most frequent cause of pneumonia, which can also come from the environment, the respiratory tract, or the GI tract. Pneumonia can also be caused by fungi, although less frequent. The environment, the GI tract, and the respiratory tract are just a few places where fungi can come from. An antiviral drug called ribavirin is used to treat pneumonia and flu. Treatment of influenza A or B infection in adults is one of the Food and Drug Administration (FDA)-approved uses. Below are some common types of pneumonia and the viruses or bacteria that can cause them.

4.2.1.1 Pneumonia due to Bacteria

The most typical form of pneumonia is bacterial pneumonia. Bacteria generally enter the body through the mouth or nose. *Streptococcus pneumoniae, Haemophilus influenzae*, and *Moraxella catarrhalis* are the most frequent bacterial culprits. Bacterial colds often last a week or so and are mild. If left untreated, they can cause ear infections in kids. Antibiotics can be used to treat bacterial pneumonia. Penicillin, cephalosporin, and clindamycin are the most often utilized antibiotic classes.

4.2.1.2 Pneumonia due to Viruses

The most frequent cause of pneumonia in children is virus. Flu, which can be caused by influenza A or B, or a virus that creates a condition identical to it, is typically to blame. A one- to two-week moderate cold brought on by influenza is possible. Although it is typically moderate, in some situations it can be severe and cause pneumonia. Antiviral medications such as oseltamivir, ribavirin, and amantadine can be used for the treatment. Usually, treatment begins 48 hours following the onset of symptoms. Septic pneumonia is the name for pneumonia caused by these microorganisms. Sometimes, bacteria from other places, such as the respiratory tract, enter the blood. In some cases, the germs enter the body through the mouth or nose.

4.2.1.3 Pneumonia due to Fungus

In children, fungus pneumonia is rare. Typically, fungus enters the body through the mouth, nose, or respiratory system. Fungus-related pneumonia is often short-lived and moderate, lasting a few weeks to a few months. Antifungal medications like amphotericin B can be used to treat fungal pneumonia. Depending on how the virus progresses to the lungs, pneumonia symptoms change.

Pneumonia (chest illness) is caused by viruses, flu-like symptoms, chills and fever, cough, chest pain, and vomiting. For diagnosis, your medical history and symptoms will be discussed with your doctor. There will be a medical examination. Also possible is a chest X-ray by your doctor, which might be applied to verify the diagnosis or look for additional symptoms. Blood tests may be done to rule out any serious illnesses.

4.2.2 Deep Learning and Its Applications

Deep learning encompasses a set of algorithms with the capability to effectively identify, extract, and manipulate features within images. Its applications in image processing are diverse and powerful. Deep learning excels in solving challenges that traditional methods struggle with, including tasks like face recognition, object detection, and image feature extraction.

These algorithms are specifically designed to tackle complex tasks such as face recognition and object detection, which pose significant difficulties for conventional approaches. Deep learning's ability to discern and manipulate image features makes it a valuable tool in various fields of image processing. It opens up new avenues for solving problems that were previously outside the scope of traditional methods.

Deep learning techniques can be used to perform a variety of tasks, such as face recognition, object identification, and object detection. If we have a sufficient amount of high-quality training data, we can successfully use all of the aforementioned strategies. We have amalgamated the power of deep convolutional neural nets with conventional Random Forest Classifiers [5, 6]. CNN design is carried out entirely in Python with the aid of Tensorflow, Sklearn, Seaborn, Matplotlib, and Numpy.

As a result, the study we propose to perform focuses on a life-threatening condition. Consequently, we have suggested a sophisticated method of carrying out the complete X-ray detection technique using deep learning and machine learning simultaneously [7–9]. Because deep learning can be used to automate processes in the future, our suggested system can capture features that were captured during training in addition to focusing on the identification of pneumonia.

4.2.2.1 Deep Transfer Learning

Deep Transfer Learning can be used to improve accuracy on a set of data with a binary class label, where a label is assigned to a data point based on a training set of examples. The process of statistical machine learning, which is the study of the theory and practice of applying statistical methods to solve a given computer science problem, also involves optimization. This can be done by a variety of methods. In learning and inference, the objective is to find a set of weights (or a vector of weights) that will maximize or minimize the likelihood of the data under the assumption that the data arises by chance alone. Variational inference is a generalization of the frequentist concept of Bayesian inference. In Bayesian inference, the question of interest is not just what parameter values to choose, but what to set as the prior distribution on the parameters, and what to set as the likelihood function. The likelihood function is the same as in frequentist inference, but the prior distribution is different. The prior distribution is chosen so as to maximize the likelihood of the data given an unknown prior distribution. This is what the variational Bayesian does. In probabilistic graphical models, the posterior distribution of the latent variables formula_1 is directly related to their marginal distribution formula_2. In this sense, the posterior distribution is a frequentist distribution. In deep learning, researchers have open sourced the state-of-the-art algorithms for image recognition, like VGG16, InceptionV3 (as discussed in Chapter 3), ResNet50, MobileNet, and so on. Using any one of the former CNNs as the images feature extractor, along with a final stage random forest classifier, would be trained on the output feature maps of the transfer learning model. Transfer learning can always play an important role while the designed algorithm can optimize the predictions up to a great extent. So, basically in this chapter we will be seeing how we can implement the VGG16 transfer learning model that would act as the feature extractor of our pneumonia detection system, along with a random forest classifier, having the parameters optimized using randomized search cross validation for the best possible accuracy while dealing with small amount of images (generally in the range of hundreds). Our designed system was coined as it is mentioned in the title, Batch-Normalizing Deep Convolutional Feature Extracting Random Forest Classifiers (BDCFE-RFCs), that would be taking inputs as Numpy arrays of X-ray images and output the corresponding class predictions, the viral pneumonia, COVID-19 pneumonia, non-COVID-19 lung infection and normal lungs. Our proposed system is capable of working with images up to 512×512×3 dimensions, but with the increase in size of images, data preprocessing would take more time, but the standard 224×224×3 works well with the proposed designed system. In Section 4.3, we will discuss how to implement the data preprocessing function to extract the Numpy arrays of the pneumonia X-ray images of patients.

4.3 THE DATA PREPROCESSING FUNCTION CREATION

In deep learning, data plays a major role in determining the overall performance of any deep learning algorithms. The way of handling the type of data depending on the domain application is very much important when we look on hands-on research. In our case we are dealing with images of X-rays of different pneumonia-affected patients and all the X-ray images are having three color channels, notwithstanding the fact that the images look gray or black and white. The images were gathered from different open sources but no need to worry as we are going to provide the links to the respective GitHub repositories also.

In Python, we have some very useful libraries that guide us to the path of creating data preprocessing pipelines and also complicated neural networks. In data preprocessing we have basically used the Opencv, Numpy, glob, and os libraries for the complete implementation. Below is the entire Python code of how we have approached the creation of the data preprocessing function. The custom function that we have created also depends on some of the keyword arguments so as to ensure proper execution during training.

The parameters of the function are:

1 RESIZE_IMAGE_VALUE: The value to which the images must be resized for the convolutional neural feature extracting random forest classifier, the default value is 224.
2. TRAIN_PATH: The path of the folder where the training datasets are loaded; basically, this is the path where all the images are present categorically, in our case all total around 400 lung X-ray images

3. VALIDATION_PATH: The path of the folder where the validation datasets are loaded same as the former, and in our case we have a total of 240 images for validation during training.
4. TEST_PATH: The path of the folder where the final testing images are loaded and these images are never seen by our CNN. We have around 150 images for final validation.
5. IMAGE_EXTENSION: The extension of all the images that our custom data preprocessing function is going to handle; default value is a string specifying the type of extension: "png," and other supported formats are "jpeg," "jpg," and "tif", but it depends on the type of domains and datasets.
6. COLOR_SPACE_CV2: This is a parameter that must not be changed and we can treat it as a formal parameter of our function. This value specifies the Opencv library of Python, which we have used for preprocessing. To use the proper color distribution as we have three channels in our images, the value is fixed to cv2.COLOR_BGR2RGB.

So, thus after seeing and having knowledge about all the parameters that we have used to create the function, it would be now suffice for the demystification of the custom-designed data preprocessing function. The function that we have created was named the "imagesToNumpyArrayFunction" and it returns the corresponding requirements for our neural network and random forest system. Below is the code for the implemented function.

```
"import numpy as np"
"import glob"
"import cv2"
"import os"

"def imagesToNumpyArrayFunction(train_path, validation_path,
test_path, resize_size, extension_of_images, color_space):"
    "train_images = []"
    "train_labels = []"
    "validation_images = []"
    "validation_labels = []"
    "test_images = []"
    "test_labels = []"
    "SIZE = resize_size"
    "print("The Total Number of Target Classes are : {}".
format(os.listdir(train_path)))"
    "for directory_path in glob.glob(train_path+'*'):"
        "label = directory_path.split('/')[-1]"
        "for img_path in glob.glob(os.path.join(directory_
path, "*."+extension_of_images)):"
            "print("Preprocessing Training images, Please
            wait ")"
            "img = cv2.imread(img_path, cv2.IMREAD_COLOR)"
            "img = cv2.resize(img, (SIZE, SIZE))"
            "img = cv2.cvtColor(img, color_space)"
            "train_images.append(img)"
            "train_labels.append(label)"
```

```
    "train_images_numpy_array = np.array(train_images)"
    "train_labels_numpy_array = np.array(train_labels)"
    "for directory_path in glob.glob(validation_path+'*'):"
         "val_label = directory_path.split("/")[-1]"
         "for img_path in glob.glob(os.path.join(directory_
path, "*."+extension_of_images)):"
              "print("Preprocessing Validation Imges, Please
              wait")"
              "img = cv2.imread(img_path, cv2.IMREAD_COLOR)"
              "img = cv2.resize(img, (SIZE, SIZE))"
              "img = cv2.cvtColor(img, color_space)"
              "validation_images.append(img)"
              "validation_labels.append(val_label)"
  "validation_images_numpy_array = np.array (validation_images)"
  "validation_labels_numpy_array = np.array(validation_labels)"
  "for directory_path in glob.glob(test_path+'*'):"
       "test_label = directory_path.split("/")[-1]"
       "for img_path in glob.glob(os.path.join(directory_
path, "*."+extension_of_images)):"
              "print("Preprocessing testing images, Please
wait")"
              "img = cv2.imread(img_path, cv2.IMREAD_COLOR)"
              "img = cv2.resize(img, (SIZE, SIZE))"
              "img = cv2.cvtColor(img, color_space)"
              "test_images.append(img)"
              "test_labels.append(test_label)"
    "test_images_numpy_array = np.array(test_images)"
    "test_labels_numpy_array = np.array(test_labels)"

    "return (train_images_numpy_array,
    validation_images_numpy_array,test_images_numpy_array,
    train_labels_numpy_array, validation_labels_numpy_array,
    test_labels_numpy_array, test_labels)"

  "RESIZE_IMAGE_VALUE = 224"
  "TRAIN_PATH = "
  "VALIDATION_PATH = "
  "TEST_PATH = "
  "IMAGE_EXTENSION = 'png' "
  "COLOR_SPACE_CV2 = cv2.COLOR_BGR2RGB"

  "(X_train, X_validation, X_test,
  y_train, y_validation, y_test,
  test_labels) = imagesToNumpyArrayFunction(TRAIN_PATH,
                                            VALIDATION_PATH,
                                            TEST_PATH,
                                            RESIZE_IMAGE_VALUE,
                                            IMAGE_EXTENSION,
                                            COLOR_SPACE_CV2)"
```

Thus, we have seen how the data preprocessing function looks like and with the help of this data preprocessing function, our AI system of CNN and random forest classifier will be getting the required data for the training and validation. The output of the data preprocessing function is corresponding Numpy arrays that would be used for training and testing. The shapes of the Numpy arrays were found to be very small as compared to traditional deep learning approaches, but in our proposed way, the application of a CNN as the feature extractor can solve the problem of feature selection and standardization.

The way in which CNNs operate on images is more complicated, which needs to be discussed in detail, but we have discussed more topics regarding the CNN in previous chapters. Therefore, keeping it aside for a moment, we can consider a CNN as a black box that is capable of performing image classification on a very large scale of data, particularly images.

The system we've developed for pneumonia detection combines a Deep Convolutional Neural Network (DCNN) as the primary feature extractor and a random forest classifier as the final stage classifier. The data used to train the random forest classifier is extracted from the final layer of our CNN. The DCNN is capable of reducing image dimensions while increasing the number of feature maps or channels. The system requires images to be reshaped to 224×224×3 pixels, resulting in an overall dataset size of [N, 224, 224, 3], with N representing the batch size.

Through data preprocessing, all images are resized to these specific dimensions, ensuring alignment and improving performance. The training dataset has dimensions [400, 224, 224, 3], followed by the validation dataset with dimensions [250, 224, 224, 3], and finally the testing dataset with dimensions [150, 224, 224, 3].

We also experimented with images of varying sizes, such as 200×200×3, 300×300×3, 412×412×3, 512×480×3, and others. The DCNN performed well with these images, with adjustments made to the number of filters in the convolutional layers. For instance, we used 20 convolution filters for the 200×200×3 size. We also tested different filter numbers for the 512×480×3 size, achieving successful results. In addition, we compared DCNN results to traditional methods using three different datasets: UCF-101, CIFAR-10, and Caltech-101. Our experiments involved both a "joint training" method and the classical method, with "joint training" involving training the neural network first on one dataset, then combining it with another dataset for further training. DCNN consistently outperformed classical methods on all three datasets.

Moreover, increasing the number of filters in the deep convolutional layers improved performance, particularly on the CIFAR-10 datasets. These results highlight the effectiveness of DCNN for object recognition tasks in machine learning and computer vision applications, including self-driving cars and medical image analysis.

An important aspect of our proposed Deep Convolutional Feature Extracting Random Forest Classifier is the custom normalization and standardization layer block used within the system's internal convolutional layers. This block incorporates batch normalization and conditional dropout to prevent overfitting during initial training, given the limited number of images, often in the hundreds. Our focus is primarily on the application of deep learning integrated with machine learning using small-scale, high-quality datasets. We also demonstrate the transfer learning approach using VGG16 as a convolutional feature extractor, but our custom-designed DCNN feature extractor outperforms the VGG16-Random Forest System.

4.4 THE VGG16 ARCHITECTURE

In deep learning, the most beautiful architecture that has ever been created was the VGG16 architecture (VGG stands for the Visual Graphics Group). The network was a fully CNN that was able to perform multi-class classification in the ImageNet competition that was held at that time for performing image recognition tasks.

The VGG16 architecture as depicted in Figure 4.2 was able to improve the accuracy rate of the ImageNet competition from ~ 75% to ~ 93% after the submission of the VGG16 network. The VGG16 network was trained with a huge amount of labeled data that was provided by the ImageNet organization, the training process took more than three weeks to complete, and the size of the dataset was in the range of hundreds of millions of images.

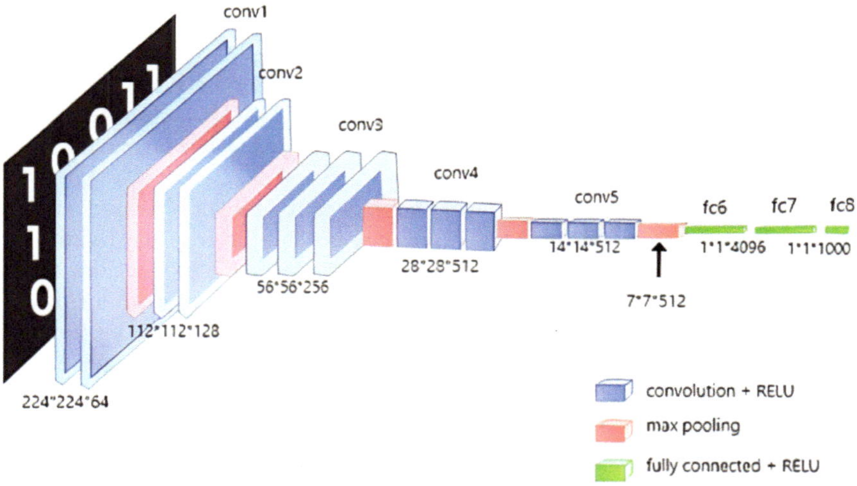

FIGURE 4.2 The VGG16 convolutional neural network.

The architecture of the VGG16 neural network was based on the CNN, and it had five different layers:

- 2D – Convolution Layer
- 2D – Max Pooling Layer
- 2D – Convolution Layer
- 2D – Max Pooling layer
- 2D – Fully Connected Layer

The convolution layers were able to learn feature maps for the input data, and the max pooling layers were able to down-sample the feature maps that were generated by the convolution layers. The fully connected layer was in charge of data classification, and the output of the fully connected layer was a vector containing the probabilities for each class of each image. Because of the architecture and the massive amount of labeled data that it was able to train, the VGG16 neural network was able to achieve such a high level of accuracy.

The design of the VGG16 model inspired the development of many other complex image recognition models, as we saw in Chapter 3 with the Inception V3 network, which is somewhat inspired by the way the VGG16 works. The combination of convolutional layers and max pooling layers, as proposed by VGG, results in a better understanding of hidden features in the provided images. The VGG16's input layer requires 224×224×3 images in batches of *N*, where *N* is the total number of images to be trained.

The output of the VGG16 has around 1,000 hidden neurons activated by the Softmax Activation function so as to ensure multi-class classification by means of probability distributions. This approach can also be found in Inception V3. Inception V3 is the new version of the Inception Architecture, and it was the winner of the ImageNet Challenge in 2015. The network was actually the first to reach a classification accuracy of more than 97% in the ImageNet challenge.

The Inception V3 architecture was based on the VGG16 architecture, but with some changes and additions. The difference between the VGG16 architecture and the Inception V3 architecture is that Inception V3 architecture has five layers and is fully convolutional.

The convolution layer is the first layer, the max pooling layer is the second layer, the convolution layer is the third layer, the max pooling layer is the fourth layer, and the fully connected layer is the last layer. Because of the architecture and the large amount of labeled data that it could train with, the Inception V3 architecture was able to perform data classification. The VGG16 architecture also inspired their own custom enhancements, such as increasing layer counts to ensure greater depth of the existing VGG16 model. VGG19 was the next resolution to outperform VGG16, effectively replacing the previous state of the art.

The VGG19 architecture is a new version of the VGG16 architecture that improved the Imagenet competition's accuracy rate from 93% to 98.6%. The VGG19 architecture is a fully CNN that is based on the Inception V3 architecture. It has seven layers and some similarities, but also some differences with the Inception V3 architecture. The convolution layer is the first layer, the max pooling layer is the second layer, and the convolution layer is the third layer. The batch normalizations layer is the fourth layer, the convolution layer is the fifth layer, the max pooling layer is the sixth layer, and the fully connected layer is the final layer. The VGG19 architecture was able to perform data classification because of the architecture, and because of the huge amount of labeled data that it was able to train with.

Thus, one constant in the application of CNNs to image classification tasks is that the amount of training data required for better results must be exponentially large. Imagenet itself contains approximately 20 million images classified into 1,000 different classes. In this chapter, we used Python and Tensorflow to build an amazing compound architecture with the VGG16 and random forest classifier. The VGG16 was used in transfer learning techniques with Tensorflow, as well as in the creation of the random forest classifier in Python. We have also provided the necessary code examples for creating the entire proposed system for pneumonia detection.

During the training of the entire neural network, VGG16 was used directly without any image training. Because VGG16 was trained on Imagenet data, it can capture image feature information; therefore, using transfer learning with pre-trained weights can solve our problem. Furthermore, we have developed our own custom DCNN that can extract image features. However, when using our very own customized CNNs, the training must be done concurrently. Because VGG16 was a cutting-edge image classification algorithm, we could expect the former to be more accurate in detecting pneumonia, but the results that we obtained were also quite impressive.

Some of different models that can also perform very well are listed here.

1. InceptionV3-Random-Forest Classifier (InceptionV3 + Random-Forest Classifier)
2. ResNet[n]-Random-Forest Classifier (Residual Networks + Random-Forest Classifier)
3. VGG19-Extra-Trees Classifier (VGG19 + Extra-Trees-Classifier)
4. VGG16-Extra-Trees Classifier (VGG16 + Extra-Trees-Classifier)
5. Xception-Random-Forest Classifier (Xception + Random-Forest Classifier)
6. Mobile-Random-Forest Classifier (MobileNet + Random-Forest Classifier)
7. VGG16-Support Vector Classifier (VGG19 + Support Vector Classifier)

4.5 OPTIMIZATION USING THE NESTEROV'S ADAPTIVE MOMENTS OPTIMIZATION ALGORITHM (NADAM OPTIMIZER)

The proposed Custom DCNN-Random-Forest Classifier System utilizes the NADAM Optimizer to minimize the loss function during the model training phase. Here's a comprehensive description of the optimization algorithm (NADAM) and its application in the system:

- Optimization algorithm (NADAM): NADAM stands for combining two optimization techniques—adaptive moments optimization (ADAM) and Nesterov accelerated gradient (NAG) optimization. The combination is designed in such a way that the resulting vectorial operation is equivalent to ADAM.
- Training Phase: Only the training phase of the DCNN requires the use of an optimizer. During training, the model learns from the data and adjusts its internal parameters to minimize a defined loss function. The optimizer plays a crucial role in this process by updating the model's parameters to minimize the loss.
- Pre-trained Weights: Alternatively, if you want to avoid the training process, you can use pre-trained weights provided by Tensorflow or another source. Pre-trained weights are learned from a large dataset and can be fine-tuned for specific tasks, saving time and computational resources.
- Training for Better Predictions: When developing a custom model, training is essential to achieve better predictions. Optimization techniques like NADAM are employed to update the model's parameters iteratively, moving toward a state where the loss is minimized.

- NADAM Optimizer: The NADAM Optimizer combines the benefits of ADAM and NAG techniques. It is used to adjust the model's parameters during training to minimize the loss function. This optimizer offers a balance between fast convergence and stable optimization.
- Hyperparameter Tuning: In practice, minor hyperparameter changes may be made to the NADAM Optimizer to fine-tune its performance for a specific problem or dataset. These changes can impact the convergence speed and the quality of the final model.

Overall, the NADAM Optimizer is employed during the training phase of the Custom DCNN-Random-Forest Classifier System to ensure that the model learns from the data and makes better predictions. It combines elements from ADAM and NAG to provide an efficient and effective optimization process.

$$\tilde{\theta} = \theta_t + \alpha v_t$$

$$g_{NAG} = \frac{1}{n}\sum_{i=1}^{n} \nabla_\theta \mathcal{L}\left(x^{(i)}, y^{(i)}, \tilde{\theta}\right)$$

After that, we compute the update rule using the gradients of the interim parameters

$$v_{t+1} = \alpha v_t - \eta g_{NAG}$$

$$\theta_{t+1} = \theta_t + v_{t+1}$$

It's evident that we apply momentum to the parameters twice—once to calculate the interim parameter and then to establish the update rule. To integrate NAG into the Adam optimizer, we need to adapt this process with the following formulation, which will be implemented within our Deep Convolutional Feature Extracting Neural Network System.

$$\begin{aligned} g_t &= \frac{1}{n}\Sigma_{i=1}^{n} \nabla_\theta \mathcal{L}\left(x^{(i)}, y^{(i)}, \theta_t\right) \\ m_t &= \rho_1 m_{t-1} - \eta g_t \\ \bar{m}_t &= \rho_1 m_t - \eta g_t \\ \theta_{t+1} &= \theta_t + \bar{m}_t \end{aligned}$$

We've adjusted the notation to align with the Adam optimizer's conventions. In this updated time-step update rule, we observe that it incorporates both the current gradient (gt) and the momentum vector of the next time-step (mt). With this modified NAG update rule, momentum is applied only once in the update process. To simplify comprehension, we have maintained a constant value of 1 throughout the training, instead of employing a warming schedule as recommended by the original author. This update rule bridges the gap between our revised NAG approach and the Classical Momentum (CM) method.

$$\theta_{t+1} = \theta_t + m_t$$

$$\theta_{t+1} = \theta_t + \rho_1 m_{t-1} - \eta g_t$$

To address the independence of the second term on the right-hand side from the current gradient, we employ Nesterov's technique to make modifications. This results in the update rule for the adapted NAG.

$$\theta_{t+1} = \theta_t + \rho_1 \left(\rho_1 m_{t-1} - \eta g_t\right) - \eta g_t$$

$$\theta_{t+1} = \theta_t + \rho_1 m_t - \eta g_t$$

$$\theta_{t+1} = \theta_t + \bar{m}_t$$

Now, recall Adam's update rule without the bias correction, and the operation of NADAM begins here.

$$\theta_{t+1} = \theta_t - \eta \cdot \frac{m_t}{\sqrt{v_t + \varepsilon}}$$

Now we will see the advancement of m_t in the optimization framework as in the CM to form the preliminary interpretation for the system's weights update rule.

$$\theta_{t+1} = \theta_t - \eta \cdot \frac{\rho_1 m_{t-1} + \left(1 - \rho_1\right) g_t}{\sqrt{v_t + \varepsilon}}$$

$$\theta_{t+1} = \theta_t - \eta \cdot \frac{\rho_1 m_{t-1}}{\sqrt{v_t + \varepsilon}} - \eta \cdot \frac{\left(1 - \rho_1\right) g_t}{\sqrt{v_t + \varepsilon}}$$

Because v_t is dependent on g_t, we couldn't directly apply Nesterov's technique to the second term on the right-hand side. As a result, the entire algorithm remains unchanged from what the authors proposed in their paper.

But if we recall, the term v_t was computed by: -$v_t = \rho_2 v_{t-1} + \left(1 - \rho_2\right) g_t^2$.

Because ρ_2 is usually set to be very large, the difference between v_t and v_t–1 will be small. So, without sacrificing too much precision, we can write the entire formulation that will lead us to the Nesterov's Accelerated Adaptive Moments also known as NADAM (NAG + ADAM) optimizer, which will serve as the main component of our convolutional feature extracting neural network system.

$$\theta_{t+1} = \theta_t - \eta \cdot \frac{\rho_1 m_{t-1}}{\sqrt{v_{t-1} + \varepsilon}} - \eta \cdot \frac{\left(1 - \rho_1\right) g_t}{\sqrt{v_t + \varepsilon}}$$

Now we can implement Nesterov's technique to the above equation and easily obtain NADAM optimizer for the system.

$$\theta_{t+1} = \theta_t - \eta \cdot \frac{\rho_1\left(\rho_1 m_{t-1} + (1-\rho_1) g_t\right)}{\sqrt{\left(\rho_2 v_{t-1} + (1-\rho_2) g_t^2\right) + \varepsilon}} - \eta \cdot \frac{(1-\rho_1) g_t}{\sqrt{v_t} + \varepsilon}$$

$$\theta_{t+1} = \theta_t - \eta \cdot \frac{\rho_1 m_t}{\sqrt{v_t} + \varepsilon} - \eta \cdot \frac{(1-\rho_1) g_t}{\sqrt{v_t} + \varepsilon}$$

$$\theta_{t+1} = \theta_t - \eta \cdot \frac{\left(\rho_1 m_t + (1-\rho_1) g_t\right)}{\sqrt{v_t} + \varepsilon} \theta_{t+1} = \theta_t - \eta \cdot \frac{\bar{m}_t}{\sqrt{v_t} + \varepsilon}$$

$$\begin{aligned}
m_t &= \rho_1 m_{t-1} + (1-\rho_1) g_t \\
v_t &= \rho_2 v_{t-1} + (1-\rho_2) g_t^2 \\
\hat{m}_t &= \frac{m_t}{1-\rho_1^t} \\
\hat{v}_t &= \frac{v_t}{1-\rho_2^t} \\
\bar{m}_t &= \rho_1 \hat{m}_t + (1-\rho_1) g_t \\
\theta_{t+1} &= \theta_t - \eta \cdot \frac{\bar{m}_t}{\sqrt{\hat{v}_t} + \varepsilon}
\end{aligned}$$

4.5.1 The Final Formulation of NADAM Optimization Algorithm

Note: In the entire description and working of NADAM optimizer, we used two terms, ρ_1 and ρ_2, which is nothing but the same values that we used during the Adam optimization algorithm and those two terms ρ_1 and ρ_2 are just an alias for β_1 and β_2.

$$\frac{\text{NADAM}\left(I_t, \alpha_t, \beta_1, \beta_2, \epsilon\right)}{m_0 = 0, v_0 = 0}$$

$$m_{t+1} = \beta_1 m_t + (1-\beta_1) \nabla \ell(\theta_t)$$

$$v_{t+1} = \beta_2 v_t + (1-\beta_2) \nabla \ell(\theta_t)^2$$

$$b_{t+1} = \frac{\sqrt{1-\beta_2^{t+1}}}{1-\beta_1^{t+1}}$$

$$\theta_{t+1} = \theta_t - \alpha_t \frac{\beta_1 m_{t+1} + (1-\beta_1) \nabla \ell(\theta_t)}{\sqrt{v_{t+1}} + \epsilon} b_{t+1}$$

As a result, the NADAM optimizer is critical in minimizing the overall loss function generated by the convolutional feature extracting neural network; in our case, we are attempting to minimize the cross-entropy error for each image and its corresponding class predictions. SGD with momentum and learning rate decay regularization, Adamax optimizer, Adadelta optimizer, and our very old Adam optimizer are some of the suggested optimization techniques if we want to use some different optimization techniques. In this chapter we are going to see how we have utilized the entire concept just by writing a function that would help us to create our very own custom neural network and also the way in which we have approached the problem of identifying lung pneumonia categories just by using the respective X-ray images. NADAM was found to be the best while training the designed feature extracting CNN. Figure 4.3 depicts the way in which we can derive different optimizers for the training loss minimization just by using the gradient descent algorithm.

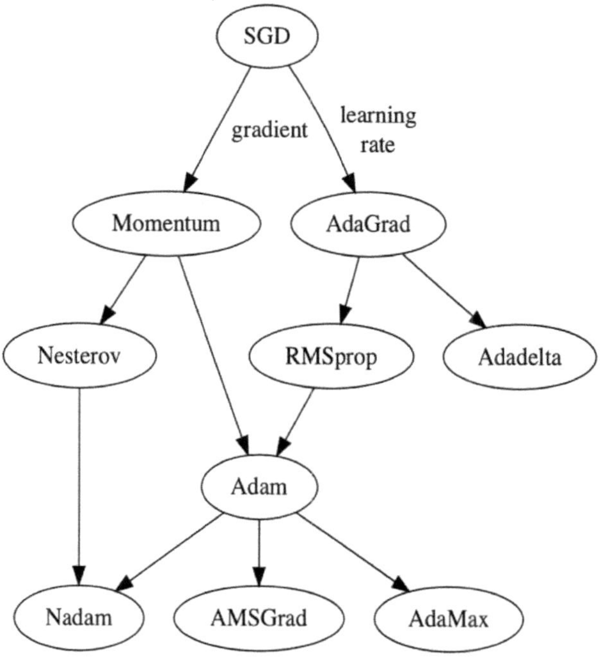

FIGURE 4.3 The way in which we can use different optimization algorithms for the training of our very own custom convolutional feature extracting neural network.

4.6 THE PYTHON CODING OVERVIEW AND GUIDELINES FOR VGG16 TRANSFER LEARNING APPROACH

In this section we will take a Deep Dive regarding the implementation of the entire system architecture in a very naive way by using certain libraries of Python. First, we will implement a way of printing the results of the former mentioned data preprocessing function that we have coined as the "imagesToNumpyArrayFunction()."

```
"def imagesToNumpyArrayFunction(train_path, validation_path,
test_path, resize_size, extension_of_images, color_space):"
    "train_images = []"
    "train_labels = []"
    "validation_images = []"
    "validation_labels = []"
    "test_images = []"
    "test_labels = []"
    "SIZE = resize_size"
    "print("The Total Number of Target Classes are : {}".
format(os.listdir(train_path)))"
    "for directory_path in glob.glob(train_path+'*'):"
        "label = directory_path.split('/')[-1]"
        "for img_path in glob.glob(os.path.join(directory_
path, "*."+extension_of_images)):"
            "print("Preprocessing Training images, Please wait ")"
            "img = cv2.imread(img_path, cv2.IMREAD_COLOR)"
            "img = cv2.resize(img, (SIZE, SIZE))"
            "img = cv2.cvtColor(img, color_space)"
            "train_images.append(img)"
            "train_labels.append(label)"
    "train_images_numpy_array = np.array(train_images)"
    "train_labels_numpy_array = np.array(train_labels)"
    "for directory_path in glob.glob(validation_path+'*'):"
        "val_label = directory_path.split("/")[-1]"
        "for img_path in glob.glob(os.path.join(directory_
path, "*."+extension_of_images)):"
            "print("Preprocessing Validation Imges, Please wait")"
            "img = cv2.imread(img_path, cv2.IMREAD_COLOR)"
            "img = cv2.resize(img, (SIZE, SIZE))"
            "img = cv2.cvtColor(img, color_space)"
            "validation_images.append(img)"
            "validation_labels.append(val_label)"
    "validation_images_numpy_array = np.array(validation_images)"
    "validation_labels_numpy_array = np.array(validation_labels)"
    "for directory_path in glob.glob(test_path+'*'):"
        "test_label = directory_path.split("/")[-1]"
        "for img_path in glob.glob(os.path.join(directory_
path, "*."+extension_of_images)):"
            "print("Preprocessing testing images, Please wait")"
            "img = cv2.imread(img_path, cv2.IMREAD_COLOR)"
            "img = cv2.resize(img, (SIZE, SIZE))"
            "img = cv2.cvtColor(img, color_space)"
            "test_images.append(img)"
            "test_labels.append(test_label)"
    "test_images_numpy_array = np.array(test_images)"
    "test_labels_numpy_array = np.array(test_labels)"
```

```
"return (train_images_numpy_array,
validation_images_numpy_array,test_images_numpy_array,
train_labels_numpy_array, validation_labels_numpy_array,
test_labels_numpy_array, test_labels)"
```

Let's us print the results that were returned by the calling of the function so as to take a look at the data set. The shapes of the data tensor are depicted in Figure 4.4.

Python Code:

```
"print("The Training dataset shape is {}".format(X_train.
shape))"
"print("The Training labels shape is {}".format(y_train.
shape))"
"print("The Validation dataset shape is {}".format(X_
validation.shape))"
"print("The Validation labels shape is {}".format(y_
validation.shape))"
"print("The Testing dataset shape is {}".format(X_test.
shape))"
"print("The Testing labels shape is {}".format(y_test.
shape))"
```

Console Output:

```
The Training dataset shape is (444, 224, 224, 3)
The Training labels shape is (444,)
The Validation dataset shape is (240, 224, 224, 3)
The Validation labels shape is (240,)
The Testing dataset shape is (150, 224, 224, 3)
The Testing labels shape is (150,)
```

FIGURE 4.4 Displaying the shapes of the data tensors (both training and validation).

As neural networks are capable of dealing with array of numbers, so the numpy arrays that we have achieved by using the data preprocessing, have values between 0 and 255 each representing individual image's pixel values. Using Python's scikit-learn library, we can solve the normalization problem of the Numpy array as well.

Python Code:

```
#Encode labels from text to integers.
"from sklearn import preprocessing"
"labelEncoder = preprocessing.LabelEncoder()"

"labelEncoder.fit(y_train)"
"train_labels_encoded = labelEncoder.transform(y_train)"
```

```
"labelEncoder.fit(y_test)"
"test_labels_encoded = labelEncoder.transform(y_test)"

"labelEncoder.fit(y_validation)"
"validation_labels_encoded = labelEncoder.transform(y_
validation)"

#Split data into test and train datasets (already split but
assigning to meaningful convention)
"X_train, y_train, X_test, y_test, X_validation, y_
validation = X_train, train_labels_encoded, X_test, test_
labels_encoded, \
X_validation, validation_labels_encoded"

############################################################
#######
# Normalize pixel values to between 0 and 1
"X_train, X_test, X_validation = X_train / 255.0, X_test /
255.0, X_validation / 255.0"

#One hot encode y values for neural network.
"from tensorflow.keras.utils import to_categorical"
"y_train_one_hot = to_categorical(y_train)"
"y_test_one_hot = to_categorical(y_test)"
"y_validation_one_hot = to_categorical(y_validation)"
```

Thus, the values that were returned by the imagesToNumpyArrayFunction, X_train, X_validation, X_test, y_train, y_validation, and y_test are now converted to the respective normalized and one hot encoded format. Thus, we can now use the Tensorflow library of Python for accessing the VGG16 CNN for performing the task of detecting pneumonia from the X-ray images.

```
"import tensorflow as tf"
"from tf.keras.applications.vgg16 import VGG16"

#Loading VGG16 model wothout classifier/fully
connected layers
"VGG_model = VGG16(weights='imagenet', include_top=False,
input_shape=(RESIZE_IMAGE_VALUE, RESIZE_IMAGE_VALUE, 3))"

#Make loaded layers as nontrainable.
#This is important as we want to work with pre-trained
weights

"for layer in VGG_model.layers:"
     "layer.trainable = False"
"VGG_model.summary()"

# Trainable parameters will be 0
"from tensorflow.keras.utils import plot_model"
"plot_model(VGG_model, to_file='VGG16-DCNN-COVID-19.png',
show_layer_names=True, show_shapes=True,)"
```

```
Downloading data from https://storage.googleapis.com/tensorflow/keras-applications/vgg16/vgg16_weights_tf_dim_ordering_tf_kernels_notop.h5
58892288/58889256 [==============================] - 1s 0us/step
58900480/58889256 [==============================] - 1s 0us/step
Model: "vgg16"
_________________________________________________________________
 Layer (type)                Output Shape              Param #
=================================================================
 input_1 (InputLayer)        [(None, 224, 224, 3)]     0

 block1_conv1 (Conv2D)       (None, 224, 224, 64)      1792

 block1_conv2 (Conv2D)       (None, 224, 224, 64)      36928

 block1_pool (MaxPooling2D)  (None, 112, 112, 64)      0

 block2_conv1 (Conv2D)       (None, 112, 112, 128)     73856

 block2_conv2 (Conv2D)       (None, 112, 112, 128)     147584

 block2_pool (MaxPooling2D)  (None, 56, 56, 128)       0

 block3_conv1 (Conv2D)       (None, 56, 56, 256)       295168

 block3_conv2 (Conv2D)       (None, 56, 56, 256)       590080

 block3_conv3 (Conv2D)       (None, 56, 56, 256)       590080

 block3_pool (MaxPooling2D)  (None, 28, 28, 256)       0

 block4_conv1 (Conv2D)       (None, 28, 28, 512)       1180160

 block4_conv2 (Conv2D)       (None, 28, 28, 512)       2359808

 block4_conv3 (Conv2D)       (None, 28, 28, 512)       2359808

 block4_pool (MaxPooling2D)  (None, 14, 14, 512)       0

 block5_conv1 (Conv2D)       (None, 14, 14, 512)       2359808

 block5_conv2 (Conv2D)       (None, 14, 14, 512)       2359808

 block5_conv3 (Conv2D)       (None, 14, 14, 512)       2359808

 block5_pool (MaxPooling2D)  (None, 7, 7, 512)         0

=================================================================
Total params: 14,714,688
Trainable params: 0
Non-trainable params: 14,714,688
```

FIGURE 4.5 The VGG model that will be acting as the feature extractor for the images.

Thus, the entire model architecture of the VGG16 is depicted in Figure 4.5, which is nothing but the console output of the aforementioned code. The VGG16 has a total of 14,714,688 parameters out of which the trainable parameters are 0 and the non-trainable parameters are 14,714,688. Thus, it proves the fact that this particular VGG model uses transfer learning.

Now let us use the transfer learning VGG model for predicting the Numpy arrays, and thus the predictions would be further provided to a Random Forest Classifier with certain trainable hyperparameters.

Python Code:

```
#Now, let us use features from convolutional network for RF
"feature_extractor=VGG_model.predict(X_train)"

"features = feature_extractor.reshape(feature_extractor.
shape[0], -1)"

"X_for_RF = features" #This is our X input to RF

"print(X_for_RF.shape)"

#RANDOM FOREST
"from sklearn.ensemble import RandomForestClassifier"
"RF_model = RandomForestClassifier(n_estimators = 50, random_
state = 42)"
```

```
# Train the model on training data
"RF_model.fit(X_for_RF, y_train)" #For sklearn no one hot
encoding
```

Console Output:

```
(444, 25088)
```

FIGURE 4.6 The feature tensor shape after the random forest classifier has predicted.

```
RandomForestClassifier(n_estimators=50, random_state=42)
```

FIGURE 4.7 The random forest classifier with detailed hyperparameter.

Thus, the outputs tell us the entire hidden story about the Numpy arrays. The VGG16 is a CNN that applies convolution operation on the images and the final output of our convolutional VGG16 was found to be a matrix of dimension [N, 7, 7, 512].

The input shape of the random forest classifier was coined as "X_for_RF" that will be having a shape of [444, 25088], where 444 represents the total amount of training samples with their corresponding 25088, which is nothing but 7×7×512, the output of the CNN, features to represent the images with. Thus, using this technique we can have an entire system where we first pass the image through the VGG16 model and then the output and feed it to a random forest classifier for the final prediction. Figure 4.6 depicts the shapes of the output after the last VGG layer and Figure 4.7 is the representation of the Random Forest Classifier with the number of internal decision trees, coined as estimators.

Below we have also provided a code by which we can find the overall accuracy of the system on unseen data Numpy arrays. In case of the random forest classifier, we are using a total of around 50 estimators with a corresponding random_state of 42, the values being decided empirically and need not be changed during the execution of the code.

Python code for determining the accuracy of the compound system:

```
#Send test data through same feature extractor process
"X_test_feature = VGG_model.predict(X_test)"
"X_test_features = X_test_feature.reshape(X_test_feature.
shape[0], -1)"

#Now predict using the trained RF model.
"prediction_RF = RF_model.predict(X_test_features)"
#Inverse le transform to get original label back.
"prediction_RF = labelEncoder.inverse_transform(prediction_RF)"

#Print overall accuracy
"from sklearn import metrics"
"print ("Accuracy = ", metrics.accuracy_score(test_labels,
prediction_RF))"
```

Let us also plot the multi-class confusion matrix for a better understanding of the predicted accuracy of 86% on test dataset Numpy array. Figure 4.8 depicts the final shapes of the training, validation and testing tensors for the system to work.

Python Code:

```
#Confusion Matrix - verify accuracy of each class
“from sklearn.metrics import confusion_matrix”

“cm = confusion_matrix(test_labels, prediction_RF)”
#print(cm)
“sns.heatmap(cm, annot=True)”
```

Console Output:

```
The Training dataset shape is (444, 224, 224, 3)
The Training labels shape is (444,)
The Validation dataset shape is (240, 224, 224, 3)
The Validation labels shape is (240,)
The Testing dataset shape is (150, 224, 224, 3)
The Testing labels shape is (150,)
```

FIGURE 4.8 The confusion matrix for the classification problem.

4.7 THE PYTHON CODING OVERVIEW AND GUIDELINES FOR CUSTOM DCNN APPROACH (FROM SCRATCH)

As we have clearly seen that the VGG16 transfer learning approach was able to reach an accuracy of 86% with a robust confusion matrix, now in this section we will determine the Python code for implementation of the entire convolutional neural feature extracting random forest classifiers; but during this time we would train the entire code on a heavy machine that has Graphics Computing Unit (GPU) capability or we can simply use the Google Collaboratory platform.

The imagesToNumpyArrayFunction creation for the data preprocessing using OpenCV, Numpy, os, and glob libraries of Python:

```
“def imagesToNumpyArrayFunction(train_path, validation_path,
test_path, resize_size, extension_of_images, color_space):”
    “train_images = []”
    “train_labels = []”
    “validation_images = []”
    “validation_labels = []”
    “test_images = []”
    “test_labels = []”
    “SIZE = resize_size”
    “print(“The Total Number of Target Classes are : {}”.
format(os.listdir(train_path)))”
    “for directory_path in glob.glob(train_path+‘*’):”
        “label = directory_path.split(‘/’)[-1]”
        “for img_path in glob.glob(os.path.join(directory_
path, “*.”+extension_of_images)):”
```

```
            "print("Preprocessing Training images, Please
wait ")"
            "img = cv2.imread(img_path, cv2.IMREAD_COLOR)"
            "img = cv2.resize(img, (SIZE, SIZE))"
            "img = cv2.cvtColor(img, color_space)"
            "train_images.append(img)"
            "train_labels.append(label)"
    "train_images_numpy_array = np.array(train_images)"
    "train_labels_numpy_array = np.array(train_labels)"
    "for directory_path in glob.glob(validation_path+'*'):"
        "val_label = directory_path.split("/")[-1]"
        "for img_path in glob.glob(os.path.join(directory_
path, "*."+extension_of_images)):"
            "print("Preprocessing Validation Images, Please wait")"
            "img = cv2.imread(img_path, cv2.IMREAD_COLOR)"
            "img = cv2.resize(img, (SIZE, SIZE))"
            "img = cv2.cvtColor(img, color_space)"
            "validation_images.append(img)"
            "validation_labels.append(val_label)"
    "validation_images_numpy_array = np.array(validation_
images)"
    "validation_labels_numpy_array = np.array(validation_labels)"
    "for directory_path in glob.glob(test_path+'*'):"
        "test_label = directory_path.split("/")[-1]"
        "for img_path in glob.glob(os.path.join(directory_
path, "*."+extension_of_images)):"
            "print("Preprocessing testing images, Please wait")"
            "img = cv2.imread(img_path, cv2.IMREAD_COLOR)"
            "img = cv2.resize(img, (SIZE, SIZE))"
            "img = cv2.cvtColor(img, color_space)"
            "test_images.append(img)"
            "test_labels.append(test_label)"
    "test_images_numpy_array = np.array(test_images)"
    "test_labels_numpy_array = np.array(test_labels)"

    "return (train_images_numpy_array,
validation_images_numpy_array,test_images_numpy_array,
train_labels_numpy_array, validation_labels_numpy_array,
    test_labels_numpy_array, test_labels)"
```

Let us print the results that were returned by the calling of the function so as to take a look at the dataset. Figure 4.9 depicts the shapes of the data tensors that were generated with the help of the data generation function.

Python Code:

```
"print("The Training dataset shape is {}".format(X_train.
shape))"
"print("The Training labels shape is {}".format(y_train.shape))"
"print("The Validation dataset shape is {}".format(X_
validation.shape))"
```

```
"print("The Validation labels shape is {}".format(y_
validation.shape))"
"print("The Testing dataset shape is {}".format(X_test.shape))"
"print("The Testing labels shape is {}".format(y_test.shape))"
```

Console Output:

```
The Training dataset shape is (444, 224, 224, 3)
The Training labels shape is (444,)
The Validation dataset shape is (240, 224, 224, 3)
The Validation labels shape is (240,)
The Testing dataset shape is (150, 224, 224, 3)
The Testing labels shape is (150,)
```

FIGURE 4.9 The shapes of the data tensors for the final modeling.

As neural networks are capable of dealing with numbers, so the values are between 0 and 255 pixels, each representing individual images. Using Python's scikit-learn library, we can solve the normalization problem of the Numpy array.

Python Code:

```
#Encode labels from text to integers.
"from sklearn import preprocessing"
"labelEncoder = preprocessing.LabelEncoder()"

"labelEncoder.fit(y_train)"
"train_labels_encoded = labelEncoder.transform(y_train)"

"labelEncoder.fit(y_test)"
"test_labels_encoded = labelEncoder.transform(y_test)"

"labelEncoder.fit(y_validation)"
"validation_labels_encoded = labelEncoder.transform(y_
validation)"

#Split data into test and train datasets (already split but
assigning to meaningful convention)
"X_train, y_train, X_test, y_test, X_validation, y_
validation = X_train, train_labels_encoded, X_test, test_
labels_encoded, \
X_validation, validation_labels_encoded"

############################################################
#######
# Normalize pixel values to between 0 and 1
"X_train, X_test, X_validation = X_train / 255.0, X_test /
255.0, X_validation / 255.0"

#One hot encode y values for neural network.
"from tensorflow.keras.utils import to_categorical"
```

```
"y_train_one_hot = to_categorical(y_train)"
"y_test_one_hot = to_categorical(y_test)"
"y_validation_one_hot = to_categorical(y_validation)"
```

Thus, the values that were returned by the imagesToNumpyArrayFunction, X_train, X_validation, X_test, y_train, y_validation, and y_test are now converted to the respective normalized and one-hot encoded format. Thus, we can now use the Tensorflow library of Python for the designing of the entire proposed system of convolutional feature extracting random forest classifier.

Python Code:

```
"activation = 'relu' "

"feature_extractor = Sequential()"
"feature_extractor.add(Conv2D(32, 3, activation = activation,
padding = 'same', input_shape = (SIZE, SIZE, 3)))"
"feature_extractor.add(BatchNormalization())"

"feature_extractor.add(Conv2D(32, 3, activation = activation,
padding = 'same', kernel_initializer = 'he_uniform'))"
"feature_extractor.add(BatchNormalization())"
"feature_extractor.add(MaxPooling2D())"
"feature_extractor.add(Dropout(rate=0.15))"

"feature_extractor.add(Conv2D(64, 3, activation = activation,
padding = 'same', kernel_initializer = 'he_uniform'))"
"feature_extractor.add(BatchNormalization())"
"feature_extractor.add(Dropout(rate=0.20))"

"feature_extractor.add(Conv2D(128, 3, activation = activation,
padding = 'same', kernel_initializer = 'he_uniform'))"
"feature_extractor.add(BatchNormalization())"
"feature_extractor.add(MaxPooling2D())"
"feature_extractor.add(Dropout(rate=0.30))"

"feature_extractor.add(Flatten())"

#Add layers for deep learning prediction
"x = feature_extractor.output"
"x = Dense(128, activation = activation, kernel_
initializer = 'he_uniform')(x)"
"prediction_layer = Dense(4, activation = 'softmax')(x)"

# Make a new model combining both feature extractor and x
"cnn_model = Model(inputs=feature_extractor.input, outputs=
prediction_layer)"
"cnn_model.compile(optimizer=Nadam(learning_rate=0.0003,
beta_1=0.5),
                  loss = 'categorical_crossentropy',
                  metrics = ['accuracy', 'mae'])"
"print(cnn_model.summary())"

# plot_model(cnn_model, to_file='DBN-CNN.png')
```

Console Output:

```
Model: "model"
_________________________________________________________________
 Layer (type)                Output Shape              Param #
=================================================================
 conv2d_input (InputLayer)   [(None, 128, 128, 3)]     0

 conv2d (Conv2D)             (None, 128, 128, 32)      896

 batch_normalization (BatchN  (None, 128, 128, 32)     128
 ormalization)

 conv2d_1 (Conv2D)           (None, 128, 128, 32)      9248

 batch_normalization_1 (Batc  (None, 128, 128, 32)     128
 hNormalization)

 max_pooling2d (MaxPooling2D  (None, 64, 64, 32)       0
 )

 dropout (Dropout)           (None, 64, 64, 32)        0

 conv2d_2 (Conv2D)           (None, 64, 64, 64)        18496

 batch_normalization_2 (Batc  (None, 64, 64, 64)       256
 hNormalization)

 dropout_1 (Dropout)         (None, 64, 64, 64)        0

 conv2d_3 (Conv2D)           (None, 64, 64, 128)       73856

 batch_normalization_3 (Batc  (None, 64, 64, 128)      512
 hNormalization)

 max_pooling2d_1 (MaxPooling  (None, 32, 32, 128)      0
 2D)

 dropout_2 (Dropout)         (None, 32, 32, 128)       0

 flatten (Flatten)           (None, 131072)            0

 dense (Dense)               (None, 128)               16777344

 dense_1 (Dense)             (None, 4)                 516

=================================================================
Total params: 16,881,380
Trainable params: 16,880,868
Non-trainable params: 512
```

FIGURE 4.10 The internal architecture of the DCNN for the classification.

Thus, we can see how we have implemented the entire DCNN from scratch using only Tensorflow and keras. The custom-designed DCNN has around a total of 16,881,380 parameters, out of which around 512 are non-trainable (due to the batch-normalization layer added in the architecture) and 16,880,868 are trainable as depicted in Figure 4.10. Thus, now we will look at how we have implemented the training with just some few lines of code and at last also concluded the training by plotting the corresponding training components. Figure 4.11 depicts the ongoing training of the designed system. Metrics plots are also provided in the Figure 4.12, followed with Figure 4.13 and Figure 4.14.

Python Code:

```
##########################################
#Train the CNN model
"history = cnn_model.fit(X_train,
                        y_train_one_hot,
                        epochs=100,
                        validation_data = (X_validation,
y_validation_one_hot),
                        batch_size=32, shuffle=True)"

#plot the training and validation accuracy and loss at each epoch
"loss = history.history['loss']"
"val_loss = history.history['val_loss']"
"epochs = range(1, len(loss) + 1)"
"plt.plot(epochs, loss, 'y', label='Training loss')"
"plt.plot(epochs, val_loss, 'r', label='Validation loss')"
"plt.title('Training and validation loss')"
"plt.xlabel('Epochs')"
"plt.ylabel('Loss')"
"plt.legend()"
"plt.show()"

"acc = history.history['accuracy']"
"val_acc = history.history['val_accuracy']"
"plt.plot(epochs, acc, 'y', label='Training acc')"
"plt.plot(epochs, val_acc, 'r', label='Validation acc')"
"plt.title('Training and validation accuracy')"
"plt.xlabel('Epochs')"
"plt.ylabel('Accuracy')"
"plt.legend()"
"plt.show()"

"acc = history.history['mae']"
"val_acc = history.history['val_mae']"
"plt.plot(epochs, acc, 'y', label='Training Mean Absolute
Error')"
"plt.plot(epochs, val_acc, 'r', label='Validation Mean
Absolute Error')"

"plt.title('Training and validation Mean Absolute Error')"
"plt.xlabel('Epochs')"
"plt.ylabel('Mean Absolute Error')"
"plt.legend()"
```

"plt.show()"

Console Output:

```
Epoch 1/100
14/14 [==============================] - 11s 98ms/step - loss: 17.5075 - accuracy: 0.4437 - mae: 0.2069 - val_loss: 3.6354 - val_accuracy: 0.2000 - val_mae: 0.3870
Epoch 2/100
14/14 [==============================] - 1s 39ms/step - loss: 0.9315 - accuracy: 0.6914 - mae: 0.1819 - val_loss: 8.6714 - val_accuracy: 0.2000 - val_mae: 0.4000
Epoch 3/100
14/14 [==============================] - 1s 39ms/step - loss: 0.5265 - accuracy: 0.7920 - mae: 0.1324 - val_loss: 11.9862 - val_accuracy: 0.2000 - val_mae: 0.4000
Epoch 4/100
14/14 [==============================] - 1s 39ms/step - loss: 0.3653 - accuracy: 0.8761 - mae: 0.1027 - val_loss: 13.8502 - val_accuracy: 0.2000 - val_mae: 0.4000
Epoch 5/100
14/14 [==============================] - 1s 38ms/step - loss: 0.2813 - accuracy: 0.9032 - mae: 0.0803 - val_loss: 15.7250 - val_accuracy: 0.2000 - val_mae: 0.4000
Epoch 6/100
14/14 [==============================] - 1s 38ms/step - loss: 0.1484 - accuracy: 0.9595 - mae: 0.0545 - val_loss: 16.7459 - val_accuracy: 0.2000 - val_mae: 0.4000
Epoch 7/100
14/14 [==============================] - 1s 38ms/step - loss: 0.1053 - accuracy: 0.9730 - mae: 0.0405 - val_loss: 17.4828 - val_accuracy: 0.2000 - val_mae: 0.4000
Epoch 8/100
14/14 [==============================] - 1s 38ms/step - loss: 0.0794 - accuracy: 0.9910 - mae: 0.0332 - val_loss: 17.3889 - val_accuracy: 0.2000 - val_mae: 0.4000
Epoch 9/100
14/14 [==============================] - 1s 38ms/step - loss: 0.0623 - accuracy: 0.9932 - mae: 0.0268 - val_loss: 16.7880 - val_accuracy: 0.2000 - val_mae: 0.4000
Epoch 10/100
14/14 [==============================] - 1s 38ms/step - loss: 0.0451 - accuracy: 0.9955 - mae: 0.0201 - val_loss: 16.2540 - val_accuracy: 0.2000 - val_mae: 0.4000
Epoch 11/100
14/14 [==============================] - 1s 39ms/step - loss: 0.0426 - accuracy: 1.0000 - mae: 0.0189 - val_loss: 15.2629 - val_accuracy: 0.2000 - val_mae: 0.3999
Epoch 12/100
14/14 [==============================] - 1s 38ms/step - loss: 0.0334 - accuracy: 0.9977 - mae: 0.0152 - val_loss: 14.9646 - val_accuracy: 0.2000 - val_mae: 0.3999
Epoch 13/100
14/14 [==============================] - 1s 38ms/step - loss: 0.0308 - accuracy: 1.0000 - mae: 0.0142 - val_loss: 14.2377 - val_accuracy: 0.2000 - val_mae: 0.3998
Epoch 14/100
14/14 [==============================] - 1s 38ms/step - loss: 0.0281 - accuracy: 0.9977 - mae: 0.0121 - val_loss: 12.2801 - val_accuracy: 0.2083 - val_mae: 0.3865
Epoch 15/100
14/14 [==============================] - 1s 38ms/step - loss: 0.0210 - accuracy: 1.0000 - mae: 0.0099 - val_loss: 11.1166 - val_accuracy: 0.2583 - val_mae: 0.3648
Epoch 16/100
14/14 [==============================] - 1s 38ms/step - loss: 0.0170 - accuracy: 1.0000 - mae: 0.0082 - val_loss: 10.3010 - val_accuracy: 0.3417 - val_mae: 0.3319
Epoch 17/100
14/14 [==============================] - 1s 38ms/step - loss: 0.0156 - accuracy: 1.0000 - mae: 0.0075 - val_loss: 9.7216 - val_accuracy: 0.3875 - val_mae: 0.3151
Epoch 18/100
14/14 [==============================] - 1s 38ms/step - loss: 0.0152 - accuracy: 1.0000 - mae: 0.0073 - val_loss: 9.2232 - val_accuracy: 0.4042 - val_mae: 0.2987
Epoch 19/100
14/14 [==============================] - 1s 39ms/step - loss: 0.0130 - accuracy: 1.0000 - mae: 0.0063 - val_loss: 8.8866 - val_accuracy: 0.4333 - val_mae: 0.2843
Epoch 20/100
14/14 [==============================] - 1s 38ms/step - loss: 0.0104 - accuracy: 1.0000 - mae: 0.0050 - val_loss: 8.4979 - val_accuracy: 0.4833 - val_mae: 0.2729
Epoch 21/100
14/14 [==============================] - 1s 39ms/step - loss: 0.0104 - accuracy: 1.0000 - mae: 0.0050 - val_loss: 8.1948 - val_accuracy: 0.4875 - val_mae: 0.2667
Epoch 22/100
```

FIGURE 4.11 First output of the ongoing training of the designed convolutional neural network model.

Console output for the training metrics plot:

The Accuracy Plot:

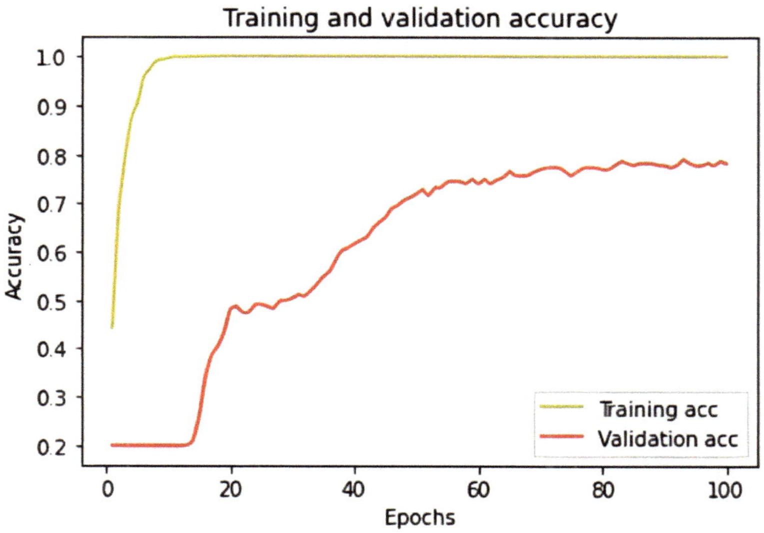

FIGURE 4.12 The Graph plot for the training and validation accuracy.

The Loss Plot:

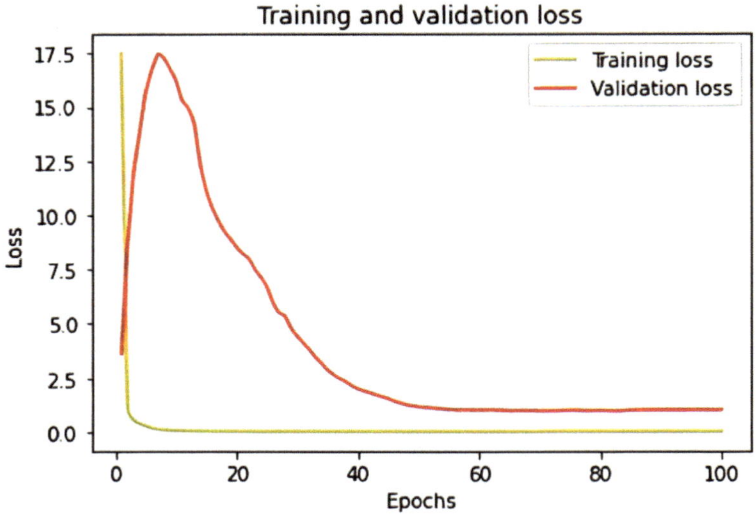

FIGURE 4.13 The graph for the training and validation loss of the model.

The Mean Absolute Error Plot:

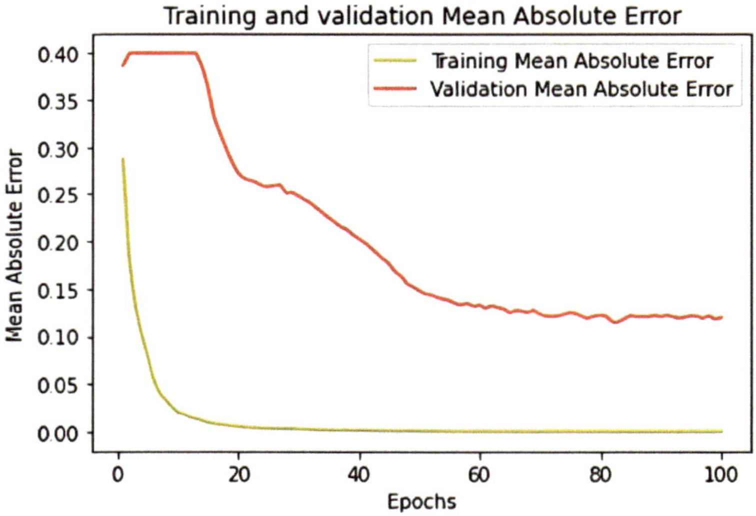

FIGURE 4.14 The graph for the training and validation mean absolute error.

Thus, by looking closely at the plots, we can conclude that though the convergence was not 100% still it can be assured that the training of the model was done perfectly. Now we will code the accuracy on test data along with the creation of the random forest classifier. But before combining the random forest, we will use the trained network to perform the predictions so as to compare ultimately. Let's use the designed CNN for traditional deep learning prediction.

Python Code:

```
"prediction_NN = cnn_model.predict(X_test)"
"prediction_NN = np.argmax(prediction_NN, axis=-1)"
"prediction_NN = labelEncoder.inverse_transform(prediction_
NN)"

#Print overall accuracy
"from sklearn import metrics"
"print ("Accuracy = ", metrics.accuracy_score(test_labels,
prediction_NN))"

#Confusion Matrix - verify accuracy of each class
"from sklearn.metrics import confusion_matrix, accuracy_
score"
"cm = confusion_matrix(test_labels, prediction_NN)"
"print(cm)"
"sns.heatmap(cm, annot=True)"
```

Console Output:

```
Accuracy =  0.7933333333333333
[[24  7  1  4]
 [ 2 17  8  3]
 [ 0  0 42  6]
 [ 0  0  0 36]]
<matplotlib.axes._subplots.AxesSubplot at 0x7f79db08a390>
```

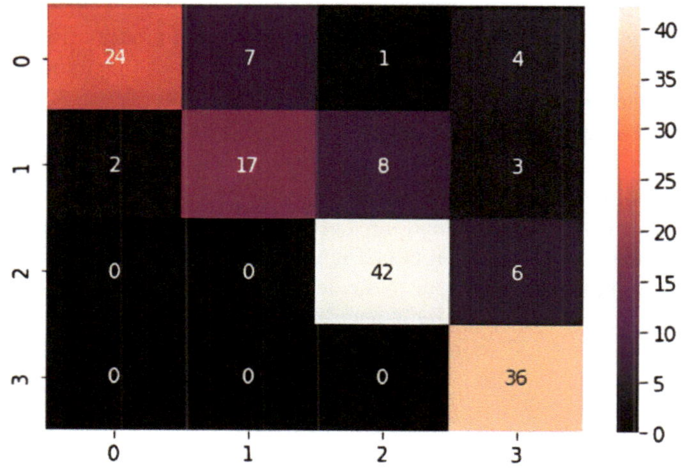

FIGURE 4.15 The confusion matrix and accuracy report for the model.

Thus, using the custom-designed trained CNN we get an accuracy of around 79 and not an average confusion matrix, as depicted in Figure 4.15, which is not that good. So let's now incorporate this trained CNN with a random forest classifier, same like the way we did for the VGG16 approach.

Python Code:

```
#################################
#Now, let us use features from convolutional network for RF
"X_for_RF = feature_extractor.predict(X_train)" #This is out
X input to RF

"print(X_for_RF.shape)"

#RANDOM FOREST
"from sklearn.ensemble import RandomForestClassifier"

"RF_model = RandomForestClassifier(n_estimators=85, random_
state=142)"
```

Console Output:

```
(444, 131072)
```

FIGURE 4.16 The feature tensor generated by the feature extractor.

```
RandomForestClassifier(n_estimators=85, random_state=142)
```

FIGURE 4.17 The random forest classifier with detailed hyperparameters.

The results clearly indicate that during the custom implementation, the outputs of the designed CNN were in the form of a matrix with dimensions [*N*, 32, 32, 128], where *N* represents the total amount of data in our Numpy arrays. The training matrix used for the random forest classifier had a shape of [444, 131,072], with 444 denoting the total number of data samples and 131,072 being the result of multiplying 32, 32, and 128. Consequently, the output of the DCNN serves as the input for the random forest classifier. In our custom DCNN and random forest classifier system, we employed approximately 85 estimators, which are essentially internal decision trees. Each of these estimators was assigned a constant random state value of 142, which remained consistent throughout the final validation process. Figure 4.16 and Figure 4.17 depicts the shapes that are generated for the system. Now, let's delve into the Python code implementation for calculating accuracy and generating the confusion matrix for the compound system, comprising the Custom DCNN and random forest classifier.

Python Code:

```
#Send test data through same feature extractor process
"X_test_feature = feature_extractor.predict(X_test)"
#Now predict using the trained RF model.
```

```
"prediction_RF = RF_model.predict(X_test_feature)"
#Inverse le transform to get original label back.
"prediction_RF = labelEncoder.inverse_transform(prediction_
RF)"

#Print overall accuracy

"from sklearn import metrics"
"print ("Accuracy = ", metrics.accuracy_score(test_labels,
prediction_RF))"

#Confusion Matrix - verify accuracy of each class
"cm = confusion_matrix(test_labels, prediction_RF)"
#print(cm)
"sns.heatmap(cm, annot=True)"
```

Console Output:

```
Accuracy =  0.88
<matplotlib.axes._subplots.AxesSubplot at 0x7f79db101ed0>
```

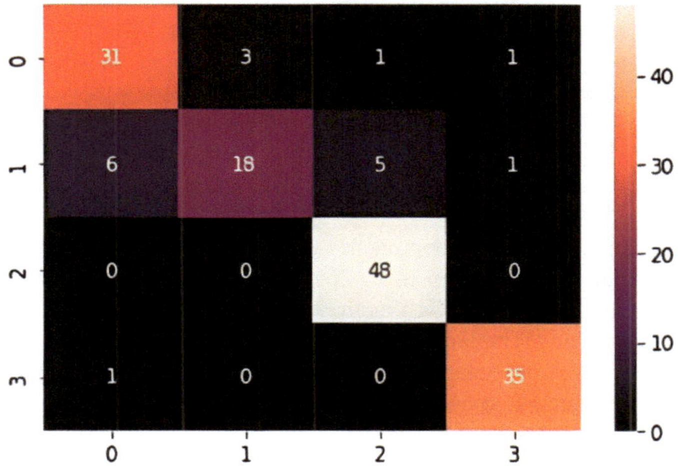

FIGURE 4.18 The confusion matrix for the trained system prediction on the unseen data.

As a result, we observed a rather surprising outcome. Our custom-designed CNN and random forest system were able to surpass the results achieved using transfer learning. When we utilized VGG16 as the image feature extractor, the accuracy reached approximately 86% as depicted in Figure 4.18. On the other hand, our custom-designed network achieved an accuracy of only 79% without the incorporation of a random forest classifier. However, when we integrated the custom DCNN with a random forest classifier, the accuracy significantly improved to 88%. Thus, our proposed system proved to be more accurate than the existing VGG16 model when dealing with domain-specific datasets for pneumonia detection. In Figure 4.19 we have provided some of the system's inferences on previously unseen X-ray images.

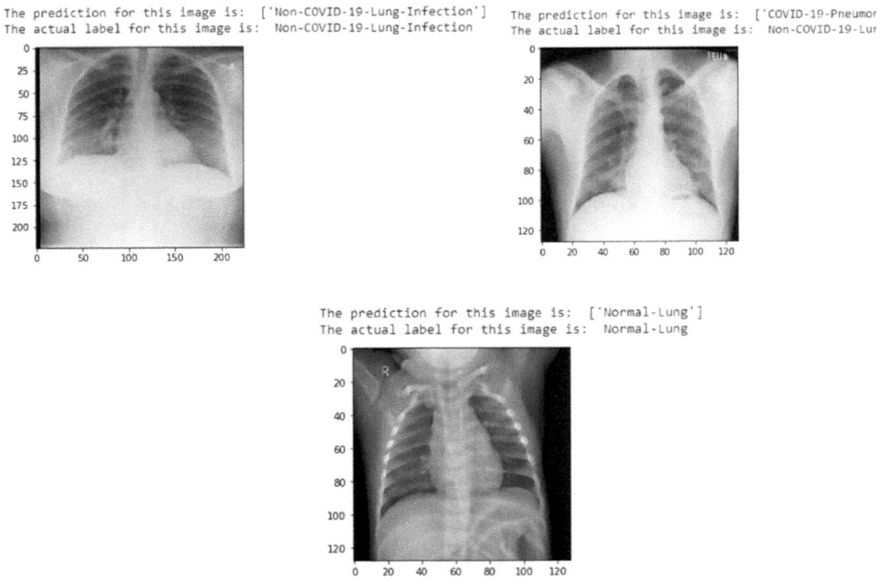

FIGURE 4.19 The ultimate predictions by the DCNN + random forest on new unseen data.

4.8 CONCLUSION

In summary, we have demonstrated two approaches to improve the accuracy of our proposed system for pneumonia detection using X-ray images of lungs. First, we employed transfer learning, utilizing VGG16 as the CNN feature extractor in combination with a specially designed random forest classifier as the final classifier. This VGG16 + random forest ensemble achieved an impressive accuracy of 86% when detecting pneumonia in unseen test images, a noteworthy accomplishment given the dataset's size.

Second, we developed a custom CNN, trained to extract features from the X-ray images more effectively. When operating independently, this custom CNN achieved a pneumonia detection accuracy of 79.3%. However, when we combined it with a dedicated random forest classifier consisting of approximately 85 internal decision trees, the system's accuracy soared to 88%. This result surpassed the accuracy of the VGG-based transfer learning system. In conclusion, despite the limited dataset size, our study demonstrates that deep learning can be applied effectively and intuitively to achieve superior results in the context of pneumonia detection. Both approaches, transfer learning with VGG16 and custom-designed CNNs, offer robust solutions. While training is necessary for creating a convolutional neural feature extractor from scratch, VGG16 eliminates the need for training as it is adept at capturing hidden features. Therefore, researchers can choose between these approaches based on their specific requirements and dataset characteristics.

REFERENCES

1. Qassim, H., Verma, A. and Feinzimer, D., 2018, January. Compressed residual-VGG16 CNN model for big data places image recognition. In *2018 IEEE 8th annual computing and communication workshop and conference (CCWC)* (pp. 169–175).
2. Abdar, A.K., Sadjadi, S.M., Soltanian-Zadeh, H., Bashirgonbadi, A. and Naghibi, M., 2020, November. Automatic detection of coronavirus (COVID-19) from chest CT images using VGG16-based deep-learning. In *2020 27th national and 5th international Iranian conference on biomedical engineering (ICBME)* (pp. 212–216).
3. Chen, A., Jaegerman, J., Matic, D., Inayatali, H., Charoenkitkarn, N. and Chan, J., 2020, November. Detecting Covid-19 in chest X-rays using transfer learning with VGG16. In *CSBio'20: Proceedings of the eleventh international conference on computational systems-biology and bioinformatics.*
4. Jiang, Z.P., Liu, Y.Y., Shao, Z.E. and Huang, K.W., 2021. An improved VGG16 model for pneumonia image classification. *Applied Sciences*, 11(23), p. 11185.
5. Chowdary, G.J., 2021. Impact of machine learning models in pneumonia diagnosis with features extracted from chest x-rays using vgg16. *Turkish Journal of Computer and Mathematics Education (TURCOMAT)*, 12(5), pp. 1521–1530.
6. Hsieh, Y.C., Chin, C.L., Wei, C.S., Chen, I.M., Yeh, P.Y. and Tseng, R.J., 2020, November. Combining VGG16, Mask R-CNN and Inception V3 to identify the benign and malignant of breast microcalcification clusters. In *2020 international conference on fuzzy theory and its applications (iFUZZY)* (pp. 1–4)
7. Menze, B.H., Kelm, B.M., Masuch, R., Himmelreich, U., Bachert, P., Petrich, W. and Hamprecht, F.A., 2009. A comparison of random forest and its Gini importance with standard chemometric methods for the feature selection and classification of spectral data. *BMC Bioinformatics*, 10(1), pp. 1–16.
8. Sylvester, E.V., Bentzen, P., Bradbury, I.R., Clément, M., Pearce, J., Horne, J. and Beiko, R.G., 2018. Applications of random forest feature selection for fine-scale genetic population assignment. *Evolutionary Applications*, 11(2), pp. 153–165.
9. Li, X., Chen, W., Zhang, Q. and Wu, L., 2020. Building auto-encoder intrusion detection system based on random forest feature selection. *Computers & Security*, 95, p. 101851.

5 An Adaptive Profound Transfer Learning Strategy for Malaria Cell Parasite Classification and Detection

5.1 INTRODUCTION

In the field of medical science and research, the majority of tests are performed by the pathologists. During a medical test, it is the pathologist who performs the test and thus results are demonstrated by doctors. Many diseases that are caused by parasites or bacteria belong to the category of medical tests, where pathologists play the primary role. Many parasitic diseases like dengue, malaria, meningitis, and so on, require at least around two to three days of incubation period and then the results are obtained. Many cases regarding malaria were investigated by doctors and some of the reports were misleading and misguiding, resulting in improper treatment of patients. So, one can never trust on tests that are performed solely by human beings as men are bound to make some mistakes during certain procedural events of malaria detection. Machine learning is that domain of mathematics and computation, where one tries to make a system that would help certain individual(s) regarding certain domains like problems. Nowadays an increase in the medical data can lead to many solutions where machine learning tends to outperform any other state-of-the-art techniques. This data acts as the main advantage regarding the experimentation of machine learning. But when data tends to increase exponentially, traditional machine learning fails to achieve the required goal.

In order to overcome this problem of data dependency, a branch of machine learning, coined as deep learning, was introduced around the mid- 1980s. Deep learning requires a huge amount of data to achieve the required goal or task. It uses the power of different types of neural networks (artificial neural nets [ANNs], convolutional neural nets [CNNs], recurrent neural nets [RNNs], etc.) to solve different data-oriented problems. Data plays a major role in deep learning and with high-quality data, deep learning can also outperform human beings. Thus, one can solely depend on deep learning for data-driven research in biomedical domain. In this chapter, we propose a deep learning intelligent system comprising different types of neural networks (CNNs) working together in an ensemble manner to perform the task of malarial cell parasite detection from parasitized cell images. The system is basically four different neural networks trained

DOI: 10.1201/9781003456476-5

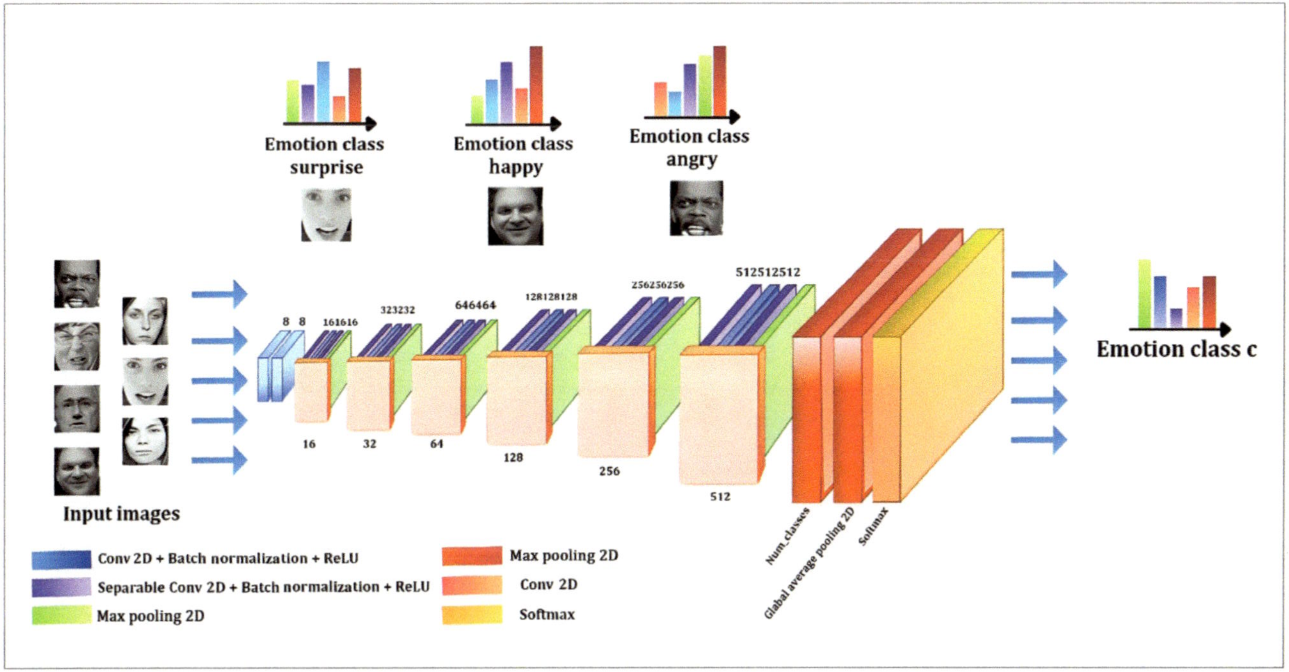

FIGURE 5.1 Demonstration of how a convolutional neural network works to perform emotion detection using images of different emotions for training.

simultaneously on the same data again and again for around two weeks. The four neural networks are CNNs, which are the best deep learning algorithm to work with when dealing with high-quality images. Inception V3 is such a CNN that outperformed many other networks in the ImageNet competition. Our proposed system's one major component is this Inception V3 network, along with three supporting CNNs: the beta-CNN, the gamma-CNN, and the delta-CNN. Thus, in this chapter, we demonstrate how the system is working to solve the task of malarial cell parasite detection just by getting trained on high-quality images for several times (Figure 5.1).

5.2 RELATED RESEARCH

CNNs can play a vital role in any big data problems where we deal with high quality of images [1]. Inception V3, a very advanced and deep CNN, replaced the state of the art in 2014 while performing multi-class image classification problems. In medical science and research, there are nowadays many domains that require some amount of automation, either mechanical automation or digital automation. When data increases exponentially, many advanced solutions can be achieved by using deep learning and machine learning [2,3]. Medical research can be sometimes very much complicated as proposed by Razzak et al. [4], and solutions to such complicated problems may lead to many innovative solutions [5]. Deep learning nowadays has found its importance in many medical research analysis challenges and the approach involves addressing these issues through various mathematical techniques applied to the relevant data, as well as employing transfer learning, as suggested by Saini et al. [6] and Zhou et al. [7]. Many papers have demonstrated how transfer learning can be used in the field of medical domain regarding images to solve some traditional challenging tasks. Wang et al. [8], Dong et al. [9] and Mednikov et al. [10] tried to solve traditional medical hazardous problems that would require some amount of digital automation. Inception V3 is the main proposed system that was utilized in the former cited papers. Using transfer learning with CNNs can be complicated to understand, yet the solution it provides always surpasses others as described by Yadav et al. [11] and Xie et al. [12]. CNNs can work in ensemble manner also to solve the directed task. Creating ensemble neural networks leads to much more complicated systems that are difficult to analyze, yet the performance tends to overshadow the complicacy. Hsieh et al. [13] demonstrated how different state-of-the-art deep convolutional neural networks can work together to solve the challenges of medical cancer. In medical research, leukemia is a very acute disease that affects many and thus Ramaneswaran et al. [14] proposed an advanced solution to this problem using hybrid CNNs and machine learning algorithms. Medical radiography also uses deep learning for digital automation as proposed by Pelka et al. [15]. Images can be of great importance while using CNNs and thus Liu et al. [16] and Li et al. [17] demonstrated how to solve challenging medical image retrieval problems. In medical science and technology, researchers are nowadays proposing many advanced architectures for solving traditional image classification and detection problems. Gaur et al. [18] and Graziani et al. [19] proposed some advanced systems of CNNs for the image analysis of certain important medical problems that would require some amount of pathological automation. Brain tumor can also be detected using deep CNNs and thus another important digital automation for pathologist is being provided in Khan et al. [20]. In medical research and science, accuracy evaluation of brain parenchymal MRI image is also an important task as presented in Kim et al. [21]. Deep learning always finds its application in medical domain [22, 23, 24] for solving many hard image classification-related problems. Lung adenocarcinoma is also an acute lung cancer problem that requires manual human interpretation. Alsubaie et al. [25] proposed such a novel system that can deal with lung adenocarcinoma growth pattern detection automation. Wang et al. [26] demonstrated how convolutional autoencoder system can be utilized for the application of denoising images of the former cited problem. Yanagawa et al. [27] and Tsirikoglou et al. [28] also demonstrated how deep CNNs can solve lung and colon cancer problems by utilizing high-quality medical analyzed images. Thus, in medical science and research, deep learning can be applied to a great extent and henceforth many digital automation systems can be possible, which can overcome certain image analysis and classification problems.

5.3 METHODOLOGY

5.3.1 The Convolutional Neural Network Using Keras with TensorFlow Back-end

With the amazing effect of convolution operation, CNNs are the kind of neural networks that can handle picture data (in the hundreds or millions of photos) in an efficient manner. Let's first study the operation of convolution before learning about a CNN. The goal of convolution is to detect the overlap between two sets of data, and the outcome of the overlap is used to determine whether the two sets of data match. Therefore, if we apply this process to two photos, we can determine whether or not there is any overlap between them. Applying this principle to an image, we can consider the entire image as one set and another image with some overlapping portion as another set. By performing a convolution operation on these two sets of images, we can determine whether there is any overlapping portion.

For example, consider that there are three sets: first set = {1,2,3}, second set = {a, b, c}, and third set = {d, e, f}.

If we want to check if the first set has any overlapping portion with the second set, then we have to form a new third set which consists of three elements from both the first and second sets. So, for this third set

we have: third set = {1, a, b, c}

Now if we perform convolution operation on these two sets, we will get a result as:

- Convolution (1st Set -> 2nd Set) = {1,0,0}
- Convolution (2nd Set -> 1st Set) = {0,1,0}

There is therefore no overlap between the first and second sets as indicated by the convolution operation result of 1, 0, 0. Convolution matrix is the name of this formula for the convolution process. There should be an equal number of rows and columns in the matrix for each sets. It is also true that the resulting matrix's dimension should equal the total of the dimensions of the two sets. To get a valid result, for instance, the second set must have at least four rows and six columns if the first set has three rows and five columns.

Let's now examine how we may apply this notion to image data.

A CNN consists of multiple layers. Let us look at a simple CNN model which consists of three layers, each layer having different functionalities.

Convolution Layer: The number of filters to be used for convolution operation is decided in this layer. There are three types of filters used in this layer, that is, 1D, 2D, and 3D filters, where D stands for the dimension of the image. Filter size is decided in this layer. Activation function to be used in the next layer is decided here also.

Sigmoid Layer: This layer can be termed as the intermediate layer, which takes the output from the previous convolutional layer and applies an activation function on it, to make the values suitable for the next layer (Fully Connected Layer).

Fully Connected Layer: This is the final layer after which a prediction is made. In this layer, a fully connected network is built where each node is connected with all the nodes from previous layers. Using this type of network, we can make predictions on the output data.

Let us see how to build a CNN for image data in Python using Keras.

We will use Modified National Institute of Standards and Technology (MNIST) dataset for this example. For this example, we will use a 2D filter and a sigmoid activation function in the convolutional layer, and a fully connected network in the fully connected layer. The model architecture will be as follows:

Convolution Layer: We will use a 2D filter of size 3×3 for this layer.

Sigmoid Layer: We will use a sigmoid activation function in this layer.

Fully Connected Layer: We will use a fully connected network with 32 hidden neurons.

We will use an input image of size 28×28.

So here is the code for this CNN in Python:

```
"model = Sequential ()"
"model.add (Convolution2D (3, 3, input shape= (28, 28),
filter=None, strides=1, padding='same', activation=
'sigmoid'))"
"model.add (Activation('sigmoid'))"
"model.add (MaxPooling2D (pool size= (2, 2), strides=
(2, 2)))"
"model.add (Dropout (0.25))"
"model.add (Flatten ())"
"model.add (Dense (32))"
"model.add (Activation('Relu'))"
"model.add (Dense (10))"
"model.add (Activation('SoftMax'))"
"model. summary ()"
```

After running the code, the following are some of the outputs which are generated on the console.

Convolution Layer:
Number of input channels: 28
Number of output channels: 32
Filter size: 3
Convolutional Padding: "same"
Network Input shape: (28,28,1)
Network Output shape: (32,32,1)
Activation function: "sigmoid"

Sigmoid Layer:
Number of input channels: 32
Number of output channels: 10
Filter size: 3
Convolutional Padding: "same"
Network Input shape: (32,32,1)
Network Output shape: (10,10,1)
Activation function: "sigmoid"

Fully Connected Layer:
Number of input channels: 10
Number of output channels: 10
Filter size: 1
Convolutional Padding: "same"
Network Input shape: (10,10,1)
Network Output shape: (10,10)
Activation function: "Relu"

The aforementioned presentation used deep learning on MNIST images, which contain roughly 60,000 training images of handwritten numbers with an average size of 28×28 and a single-color channel (black and white images). The precision of the entire system of classifying digits was the clear advantage of utilizing a CNN over any other deep learning technique. Such a CNN system utilized for MNIST handwritten digits recognition is shown in Figure 5.2.

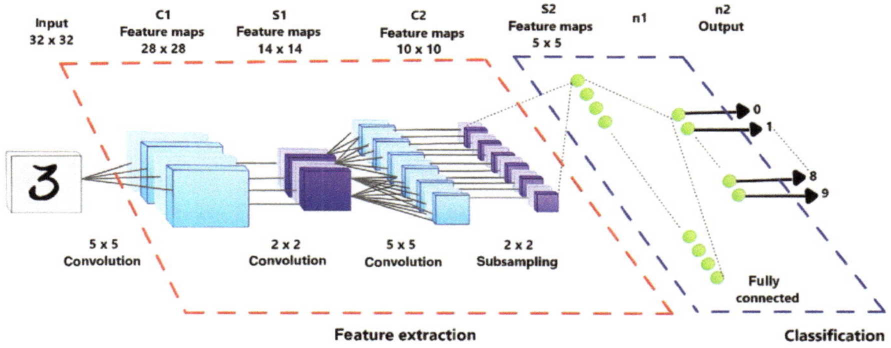

FIGURE 5.2 A CNN system for handwritten digits recognition.

5.3.2 The Inception V3 Architecture

CNNs have proven their effectiveness in image processing tasks, especially when trained on high-quality image data. Proper training can lead to accuracy levels that surpass those achieved by current state-of-the-art algorithms. Google introduced the concept of a deep CNN, specifically the Inception V3 Network, which is capable of having more than 150 layers. This deep architecture not only increases the depth of the network but also incorporates design elements to reduce the number of parameters in each layer, effectively reducing the overall parameter count.

When increasing the depth of a neural network, the risk of overfitting becomes a concern. However, Google's Inception V3 Network addresses this issue through its unique architectural components, which help minimize the number of parameters in each layer. The name "Inception" is inspired by the movie of the same name, starring Leonardo DiCaprio, which explores the concept of interconnected dreams that influence the final outcome in a unique way. Initially proposed as GoogLeNet, Inception V3 was further refined and open-sourced for transfer learning purposes.

The Inception V3 Network begins with a colored image input of dimensions 299×299×3. The image undergoes a sequential reduction in size through a series of convolutional layers: the first layer with 32 features, a size of 3×3, and a stride of 2×2; the second layer with 32 features, a size of 3×3, and a stride of 1×1; and the third layer with 64 features, a size of 3×3, and a stride of 1×1. This process reduces the image dimensions while increasing the number of feature maps. Additionally, the network incorporates max pooling layers as part of its architecture to enhance its capabilities reducing the dimensions and increasing the feature maps a bit.

The entire Inception V3 architecture is consisted of convolutional layers and max pooling layers operating upon the provided image in different stages. Inception V3 network has mainly five important parameter tuning and reducing components. Inception Block A, Inception Block B, and Inception Block C are the three main blocks for increasing the feature vector in such a way that the overall depth of the network is increased. Reduction Block A and Reduction Block B are the two components of Inception V3 that is responsible for the reduction of parameters of the supplied images. The network is a bit special when observed from the end point. The network is comprised of two different dense network classifiers: the auxiliary classifier and the main classifier. The auxiliary classifier acts like the first dream as depicted in the aforementioned movie, the outputs of which indirectly affect the outputs of the main classifier. Google proposed that the number of auxiliary classifiers can be increased depending on the problem and also the resources must be upgraded accordingly. Let us see the detailed overview of this Inception V3 CNN.

In Figure 5.3, Inception Block A and Inception Block B are shown in detail. Both the blocks accept inputs from the previous layers as four-dimensional tensors like [25000,299,299,3], where 25000 is the batch size of images and 299,299,3 depicts the image size. The concept of using multiple sized convolutional kernels simultaneously is being utilized in these two blocks.

Inception Block A is consisted of only max pooling and convolutional layers, applied upon the image simultaneously, at different stages. First, the usage of 1×1 convolution is used in a branched manner upon the same previous input. The 1×1

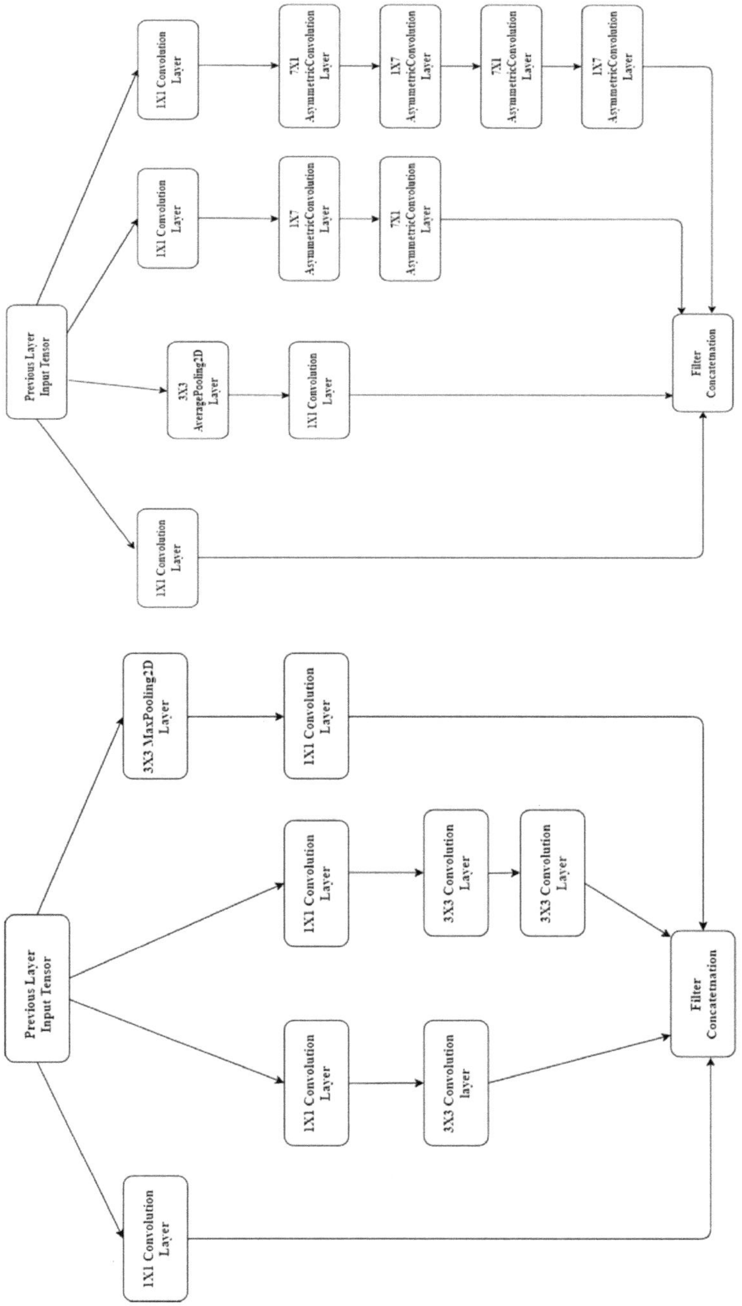

FIGURE 5.3 Inception Block A (left) and Inception Block B (right).

convolution acts like a parameter reducer and thus the entire image dimensions are reduced. The block also uses a 3×3 max pooling layer that is capable of further reducing the size and also capturing certain dominant features of the image. Convolutional layers are also used in this block but with fixed kernel size of 3×3 for increasing the feature vector and reducing the dimensions as well. Thus, all the outputs of the corresponding convolutional layers and max pooling layers are concatenated in the end and thus yielding another four-dimensional tensor, like [25000, 147,147,64], where 147×147 is the final reduced size of the tensor with corresponding 64 convolutional feature maps capturing different important features.

Inception Block B is mainly there for reducing the parameters again. This block uses the concept of asymmetric convolutions applied simultaneously on the input to the block. The three asymmetric convolutions are divided into two groups for two paths: one is followed by 1×7 and 7×1 asymmetric convolutions and the other is consisted of a repeated block of this 1×7 and 7×1 asymmetric convolutions that is capable of reducing the parameters to a great extent. This particular block uses this concept of factorizing convolutions into multiple asymmetric convolutions. In the earlier versions of Inception, this modification was not introduced and hence we can consider this as an additional improvisation to the existing architecture. This layer also takes a four-dimensional tensor as an input and finally after performing the entire procedural operations, the outputs of the respective blocks are once again concatenated.

Inception Block C is provided to the architecture just as a modification to the previous reduction component, the asymmetrical convolutions. In this particular block, the layers are mainly convolutional and max pooling, the convolutional layers are there to again reduce the dimensions and then increase the overall final features of the tensor provided as input to the block. This particular block acts like a hybrid of Block A and Block B, mainly focusing on the asymmetrical convolutional layers. In the block, the 3×3 convolutions are replaced by blocks of 1×3 and 3×1 convolutions that try to reduce the overall percentage of parameters in the block. Figures 5.4 and 5.5 present Inception Block C and how the asymmetrical convolutions are happening simultaneously.

In the Inception V3 network, the reduction of image dimensions relies on specific reduction blocks integrated into the network. Two such reduction blocks, Reduction Block A and Reduction Block B, play a crucial role in reducing the dimensions of the feature-rich output from internal blocks. These reduction blocks are strategically placed within the network after the corresponding inception blocks.

Reduction Block A employs a combination of convolutional layers and 3×3 max pooling layers to further enhance feature extraction while reducing tensor dimensions. Similar to inception blocks, reduction blocks follow the principle of reducing layer parameters to allow for deeper and wider networks. Multiple convolutional kernel sizes are utilized to capture intricate details.

On the other hand, Reduction Block B also utilizes the concept of asymmetrical convolutions to minimize the total number of parameters at the final concatenation of layer outputs. This block employs convolutional layers with max pooling at specific intervals, featuring a modification involving a 1×7 and 7×1 asymmetrical convolution block, repeated once after a 1×1 convolution. Both Reduction Block A and Reduction

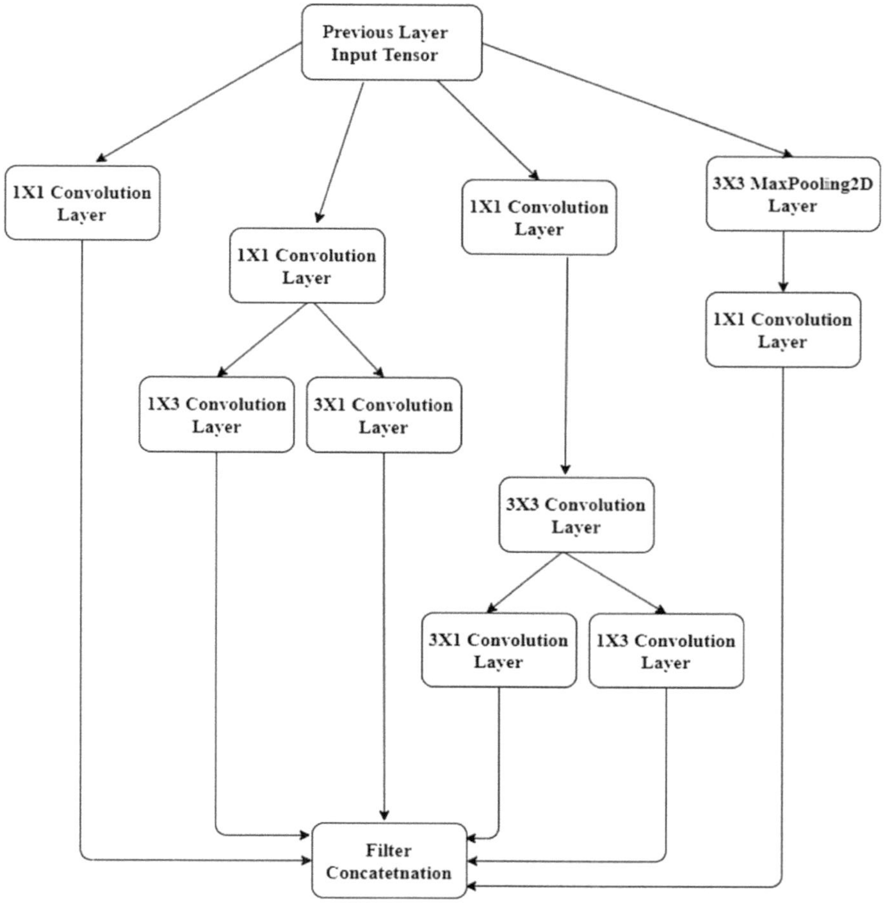

FIGURE 5.4 Inception Block C.

Block B work in parallel on their respective inputs, and their outputs are concatenated before being passed to subsequent layers.

With these reduction blocks defined, the overall architecture of Inception V3 can be structured. Figure 5.6 presents an illustration of how to design the complete Inception V3 architecture for specific problem-solving tasks. It showcases how these blocks contribute to parameter reduction and feature map expansion, enabling the network to effectively implement the concept of "Going Deeper with Convolutions."

The entire Inception V3 architecture is depicted in Figure 5.6 with all the incorporation of the blocks, the three inception blocks, and the two reduction blocks. The architecture mainly focuses on reduction of the layer parameters along with simultaneously increasing the feature maps by utilizing the reduction blocks. The Inception V3 requires inputs to be passed in dimension of 299×299×3. This input is passed on

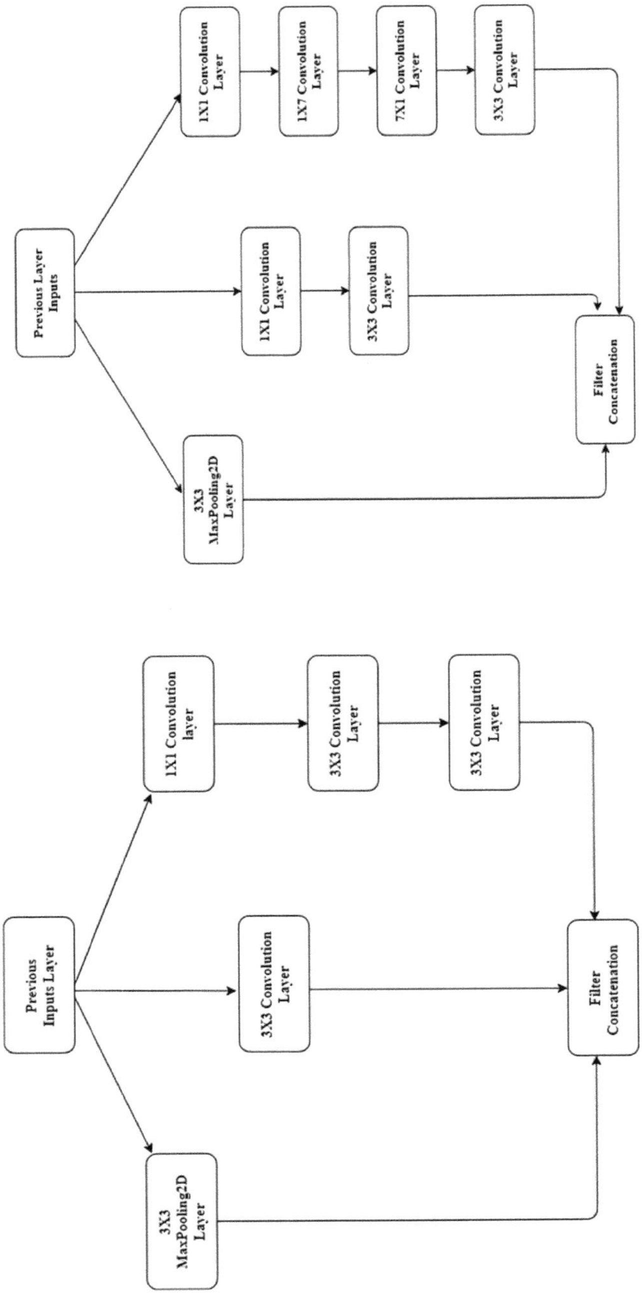

FIGURE 5.5 The Inception V3 Reduction Block A (left) and the Inception V3 Reduction Block B (right).

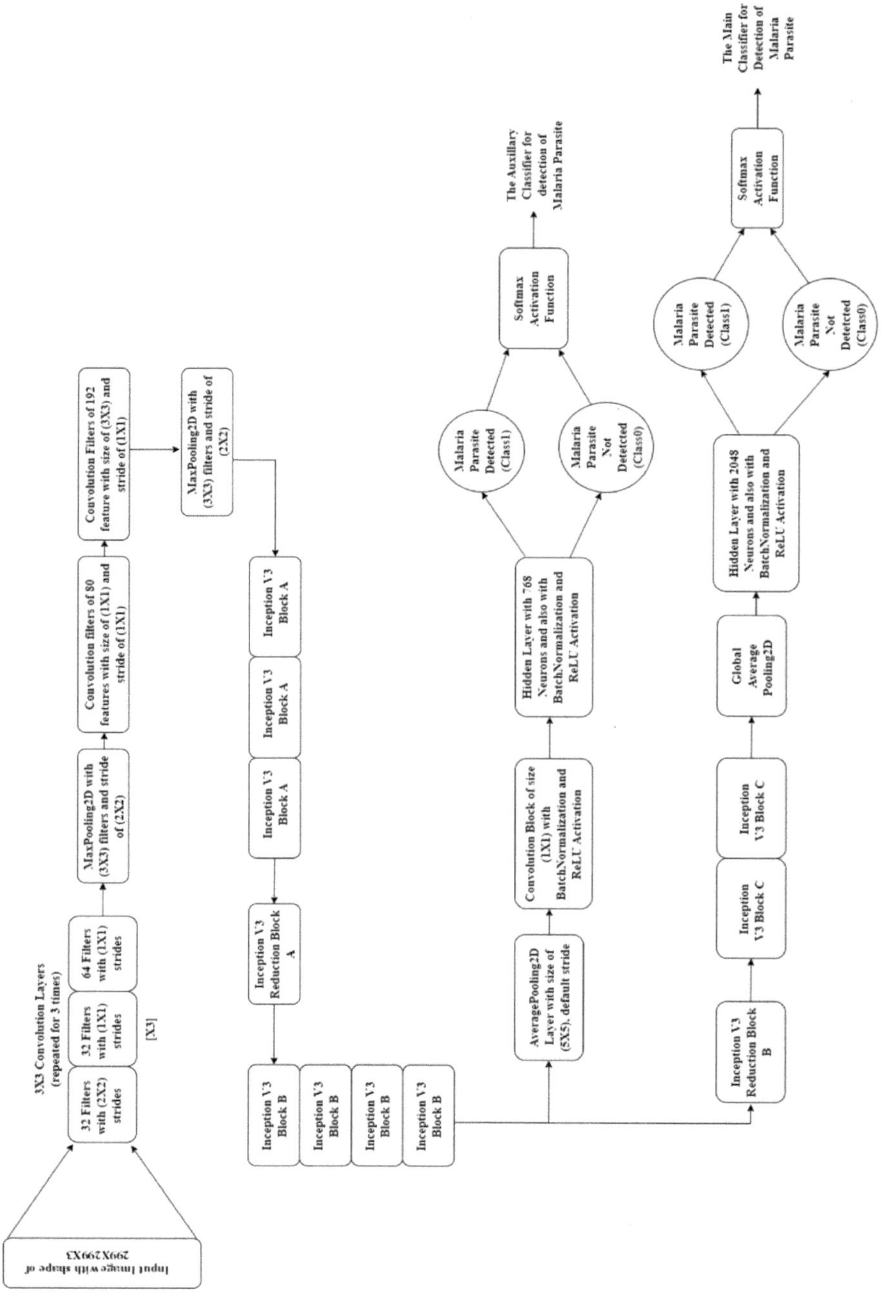

FIGURE 5.6 The Inception V3 architecture.

to the 3×3 convolutional layer blocks that encompass the reduction of dimension from 299×299×3 to 147×147×64, where 64 represents the convolutional feature maps and the dimension is getting reduced by 50%. The outputs of the convolutional blocks are then passed to the max pooling 2D layer for further reduction of parameters from 147×147×64 to 78×78×64 for going much deeper into convolutions. The output of the max pooling 2D layer is then passed to the next convolutional blocks that reduce the dimensions further and hence the entire output of the system is provided to Inception Block A which is getting repeated for four times and followed with the implementation of the Reduction Block A, which then increases the feature maps, and the dimensionality reduction is achieved parallelly.

After the data is passed and processed by Inception Block A and Reduction Block A, the outputs are then passed to Inception Block B, which is again getting repeated for around four times, ensuring further reduction of parameters and depth of the network as well. This reduction of parameters happens due to the presence of the asymmetrical convolutions applied to the data. This reduction of parameters is mainly handled by Inception Block B and Reduction Block A. The outputs of Inception Block B are then separately passed to the auxiliary path which then follows the auxiliary classifier, and the other is passed to Reduction Block B which again reduces the parameters and ensures that greater depth can be achieved by the network. Reduction Block B acts just like Inception Block B, utilizing the same 1×7 and 7×1 asymmetrical convolutions for reduction of dimensions and layer parameters. This reduction of parameters is ensured by Reduction Block B so as to make the data suitable enough for Inception Block C. Inception Block C acts like an ultimate component for reducing the parameters of the overall network and also ensures that the aforementioned system can be repeated for many more times, so as to increase the depth further and also reduce the parameters of the layers.

Inception Block C utilizes the concept of factorization into asymmetric convolutions from 3×3 to two layers having 1×3 and 3×1 asymmetrical convolutions, thus decreasing the percentage of parameters. Thus, the outputs of Inception Block C are then passed to the final classifier for the final prediction. The Inception V3 network can be considered as a way of getting very deep with convolution operations so that one can understand the different hidden features present in the provided image. The way in which the Inception V3 network works is a bit advanced but yet effective as previously when people designed very deep neural networks; the main problem that appears is the problem of overfitting and a decrease in the overall performance of the network during the validation phase.

Thus, the entire Inception V3 architecture working procedure is provided and, hence, in this work we have proposed to use this Inception V3 network along with two other CNNs that are acting to provide the Inception V3 a higher order of threshold confidence. Thus, we have proposed in this chapter how one can create an ensemble transfer learning system comprising multiple neural nets performing together during the final prediction. The two other CNNs that help the Inception V3 network are designed accordingly to match the way in which Inception V3 works and allow us to get the best predictions out from the entire system of the CNNs. The entire system is designed in such a way that the greatest possible accuracy regarding the problem for detection of malaria cell parasite can be achieved.

5.3.3 Algorithmic Approach and Working Principle of the ADAM Optimizer

Require: Step size
Require: $\beta_1, \beta_2 \in [0,1)$: Exponential decay rates for the moment estimates
Require: $f(\theta)$: Stochastic objective function with parameters θ
Require: θ_0 : Initial parameter vector
$m_0 \leftarrow 0$ (Initialize 1st moment vector)
$v_0 \leftarrow 0$ (Initialize 2nd moment vector)
$t \leftarrow 0$ (Initialize timestep)
while θ_t not converged
do { $t \leftarrow t+1 g_t \leftarrow \nabla_\theta f_t(\theta_{t-1})$ (Get gradients w.r.t. stochastic objective at time step t)
$m_t \leftarrow \beta_1 \cdot m_{t-1} + (1-\beta_1)\cdot g_t$ (Update biased first moment estimate)
$v_t \leftarrow \beta_2 \cdot v_{t-1} + (1-\beta_2)\cdot g_t^2$ (Update biased second raw moment estimate)
$\hat{m}_t \leftarrow m_t / (1-\beta_1^t)$ (Compute bias-corrected first moment estimate)
$\hat{v}_t \leftarrow v_t / (1-\beta_2^t)$ (Compute bias-corrected second raw moment estimate)
$\theta_t \leftarrow \theta_{t-1} - \alpha \cdot \hat{m}_t / (\sqrt{\hat{v}_t} + \epsilon)$ (Update parameters)
end while

Return θ_t (Resulting parameters)
}

The ADAM optimizer is merely a momentum-added RMSprop and Stochastic Gradient Descent (SGD). It scales the learning rate using squared gradients, similar to RMSprop, and leverages momentum by using the gradient's moving average rather than the gradient itself, similar to SGD with momentum. Let's examine its operation in more detail.

This optimizer computes individual learning rates for various parameters according to an adaptive learning rate algorithm. Because ADAM employs estimations of the first and second moments of the gradient to change the learning rate for each weight of the neural network, it gets its name from the term "adaptable moment estimation." In a formal way:

$$m_n = E[X^n]$$

where m = moment, X = random var iable.

Since all deep neural network's gradients are often calculated using a tiny random batch of data, they can be thought of as random variables. The first instant is the actual mean, while the second is the uncluttered variance (in which case the mean is not subtracted when calculating the variance). The ADAM optimizer uses exponential moving averages, computed on the gradient evaluated on a current mini-batch, to estimate the moments considerably more precisely. The foundational formulation from the ADAM optimizer original publication served as the basis for our suggested study. This optimization approach is used in the very first step of our proposed model, the multimodal system, which is the training of our three separate CNNs.

The basic ADAM formulas are provided below.

$$m_t = \beta_1 m_{t-1} + (1-\beta_1) g_t \; V_t = \beta_2 V_{t-1} + (1-\Delta_2) g_t^2$$

Moving averages, the gradient of the most recent mini-batch, and the newly introduced hyperparameters of the method beta 1 and beta 2 are all present.

They both have excellent default values at the beginning of the iteration, moving average vectors are initialized with zeros. Let's look at the expected values of our moving averages to determine how these values correspond to the current situation. We want to have the following property as the estimates of the first and second moments:

$$E[m_t] = E[g_t] \; E[v_t] = E[g_t^2]$$

With this situation, the parameter is also the expected value, which is surprising because the expected values of the estimators should match the parameter we're trying to estimate. These characteristics would indicate the existence of unbiased estimators if they were true. We'll see next that these do not apply to our moving averages. The estimators are skewed toward zero because we start averages with zeros.

We have also created an analytical and condensed attempt to demonstrate the entirety of the aforementioned concept. The following is the primary extension of the entire ADAM concept.

$$\begin{aligned} m_0 &= 0 m_1 = \beta_1 m_0 + (1-\beta_1) g_1 = (1-\beta_1) g_1 \, m_2 \\ &= \beta_1 m_1 + (1-\beta_1) g_2 = \beta_1 (1-\beta_1) g_1 + (1-\beta_1) g_2 \, m_3 \\ &= \beta_1 m_2 + (1-\beta_1) g_3 = \beta_1^2 (1-\beta_1) g_1 + \beta_1 (1-\beta_1) g_2 + (1-\beta_1) g_3 \end{aligned}$$

As we can see, the early values of gradients contribute less and less to the overall value as we "further" extend the value because they are multiplied by smaller and smaller beta. By rewriting the moving average formula as shown below to capture this pattern, we may arrive at the true formulation of the ADAM optimizer for our ensemble CNN system.

$$m_t = (1-\beta_1) \sum_{i=0}^{t} \beta_1^{t-i} g_i$$

Let's take a look at the expected value of *m*, to see how it relates to the true first moment, so we can correct for the discrepancy of the two:

$$E[m_t] = E\left[(1-\beta_1) \sum_{i=1}^{t} \beta_1^{t-i} g_i\right] = E[g_i](1-\beta_1) \sum_{i=1}^{t} \beta_1^{t-i} + \zeta = E[g_i](1-\beta_1) + \zeta$$

5.3.3.1 Bias Correction for the First Momentum Estimator

We enlarge the first row using our new moving average formula. Given that it no longer depends on i, we can now remove it from the sum. The formula shows the error C as a result of the approximation. The formula for the sum of a finite geometric series is all that is used in the final line.

The following will be the estimator's final formula:

$$m\hat{}_t = \frac{m_t}{1-\beta_1} v\hat{}_t = \frac{v_t}{1-\beta_2}$$

The only thing left to do is to use those moving averages to scale learning rate individually for each parameter.

$$w_t = w_{t-1} - \eta \frac{m\hat{}_t}{\sqrt{v\hat{}_t + \epsilon}}$$

Model weights are located where eta (which resembles the letter n) is the step size (it can depend on iteration). The update rule for Adam that we have utilized in our suggested work is complete. During the training of the looping DCNN and the multimodal DCNN, the ADAM optimizer is crucial. In our proposed ensemble deep learning system, ADAM optimizer reduces the loss function produced by the associated CNNs.

5.3.4 The Concept of the Ensemble Creation

With the Inception V3 network, we proposed to use two other different CNNs and the former would be working in an ensemble way during the final prediction. The entire system can be considered a group of CNNs, and the system is an automated way of determining the category to which the image inputs belong. The system is capable of performing in an ensemble way just like the operation of a random forest classifier. CNNs follow the theory of convolution and how images can be treated as a matrix of integers.

The images that we are dealing in this work are resized to a dimension of 300×300×3 such that the Inception V3 can deal with it, along with the two others as well. We have created the system in such a way that the training procedure can be minimized in time. We trained the entire ensemble system for around 75 epochs for the multimodal DCNN and 50 epochs for the looping DCNN, Inception being only trained for around 35 epochs. During the training the optimizers that we have proposed to use are Adam, with a learning rate of 0.00075, beta_1 being 0.87, beta_ being 0.95, with a corresponding epsilon value of 1.15e-07 and a schedule decay of 2.25e-08. The entire architecture of the system is demonstrated in Figure 5.7.

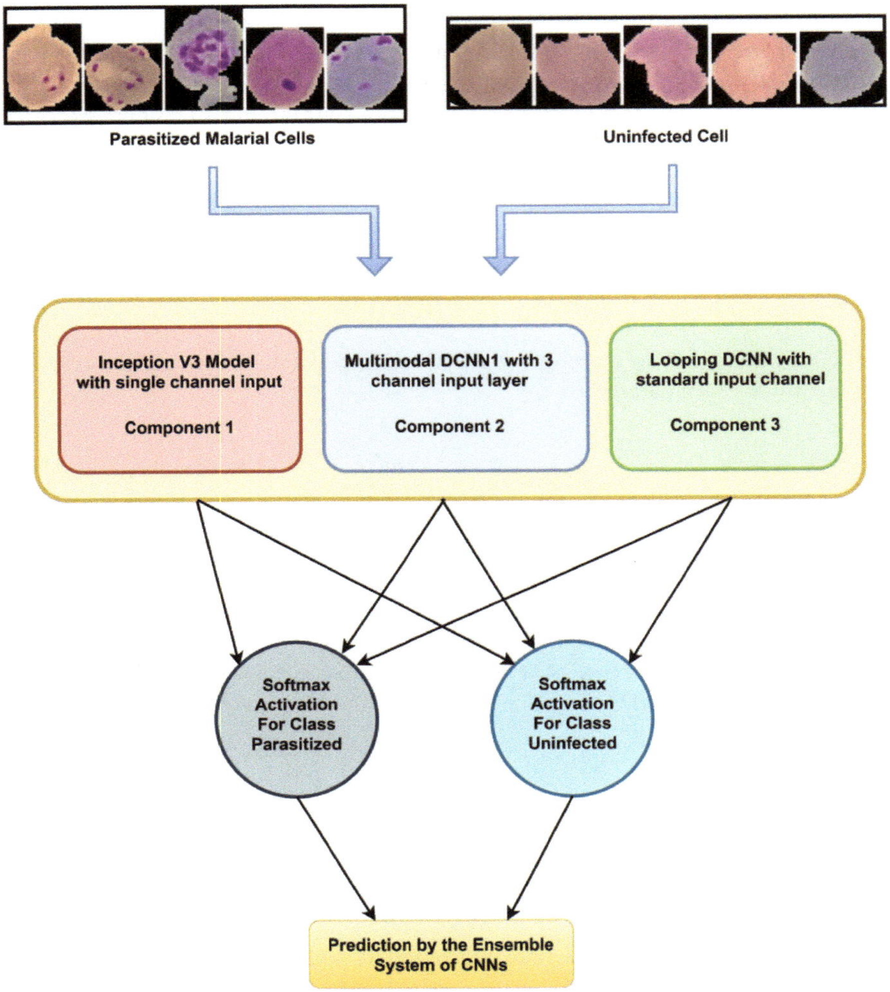

FIGURE 5.7 The entire block diagram of the proposed system with Inception V3, multimodal DCNN1, and the looping DCNN.

TensorFlow and Open-CV, which are used for both the system architecture and the image processing, are integrated into the proposed system's Python code. The multimodal DCNN and the looping DCNN are the two supports for the Inception V3 network. The multimodal DCNN is a specifically created CNN that functions with the aid of convolution operations functioning in a three-channeled manner in order to make the network broad enough to capture several features in the form of convolutional filters. Figure 5.8 demonstrates the entire multimodal DCNN in the form of blocks representing each layers along with the dimensions of the incoming inputs.

The multimodal DCNN operates sequentially and has three convolutional branches, each of which contains an input layer with the dimensions 300×300×3. As many characteristics as possible are collected using the three convolutional channels to ensure accurate prediction and identification of the input images. Using the Nadam optimizer, the multimodal DCNN was trained with a learning rate of 0.0072, 87% of beta 1 and 92.5% of beta 2, with a constant learning rate of 1.15e-08. GridSearchCV and RandomizedSearchCV are also used to tune hyperparameters.

With the appropriate Nadam optimizer and a batch of 256 images, the multimodal DCNN is trained for roughly 75 epochs, and the output graphs are rather impressive. The multimodal DCNN model validated pretty well, with a validation accuracy of 95.12% and a validation loss of 0.0752. The training accuracy was 92.75% and the equivalent loss was 0.175. Since our dataset was restricted to only 250 photos per class with a dimension of 720x480 apiece, employing more high-quality images is one way to improve the accuracy and overall performance of the multimodal DCNN (Figure 5.9).

With an impressive accuracy of 98.49% achieved by the multimodal DCNN, which was trained concurrently with Inception V3 on the malarial parasite dataset, it stands as a testament to being a deep and extensive CNN. This suggests that the multimodal DCNN possesses the capability to extract a broader spectrum of features from the images on which it was trained. Prior to undergoing multiple convolutional and maximum pooling layers, the inputs to this neural network were shaped into a 300×300×3 matrix.

On the other hand, the bimodal looping DCNN, the second component of our ensemble system, is illustrated in Figure 5.10. Operating in accordance with the principles of residual networks, it demonstrates how skip connections can be effectively employed to enable deeper neural network processing. The bimodal looping DCNN, functioning akin to a deep residual network, excels in capturing various hidden features that may otherwise be challenging for neural networks to capture at certain stages of training. Given the emphasis on deep convolutional layers, the application of residual networks holds significant value. The block diagram, along with internal convolutional dimensions, is presented in Figures 5.10 and 5.11.

The primary objective behind employing such a complex architecture is to leverage the Inception V3 concept in tandem with custom deep residual networks featuring internal connections. This architectural sophistication contributes to enhanced feature extraction and, ultimately, more accurate and robust results and also better optimization of weights during training (Figure 5.11).

Hence, the bimodal looping DCNN can be envisioned as an extensively deep and wide CNN, trained in parallel with Inception V3 and the multimodal DCNN on the malarial parasite dataset. This network achieved an impressive accuracy rate of 98.25%, indicating its ability to capture a broader range of features from the

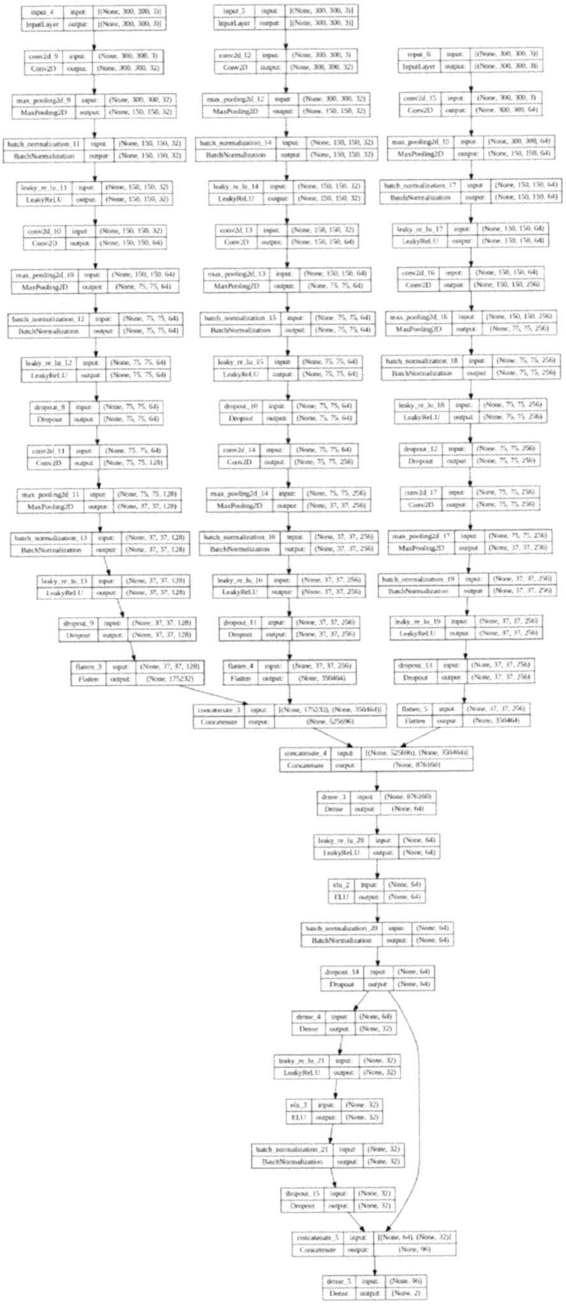

FIGURE 5.8 The multimodal DCNN (deep convolutional neural network).

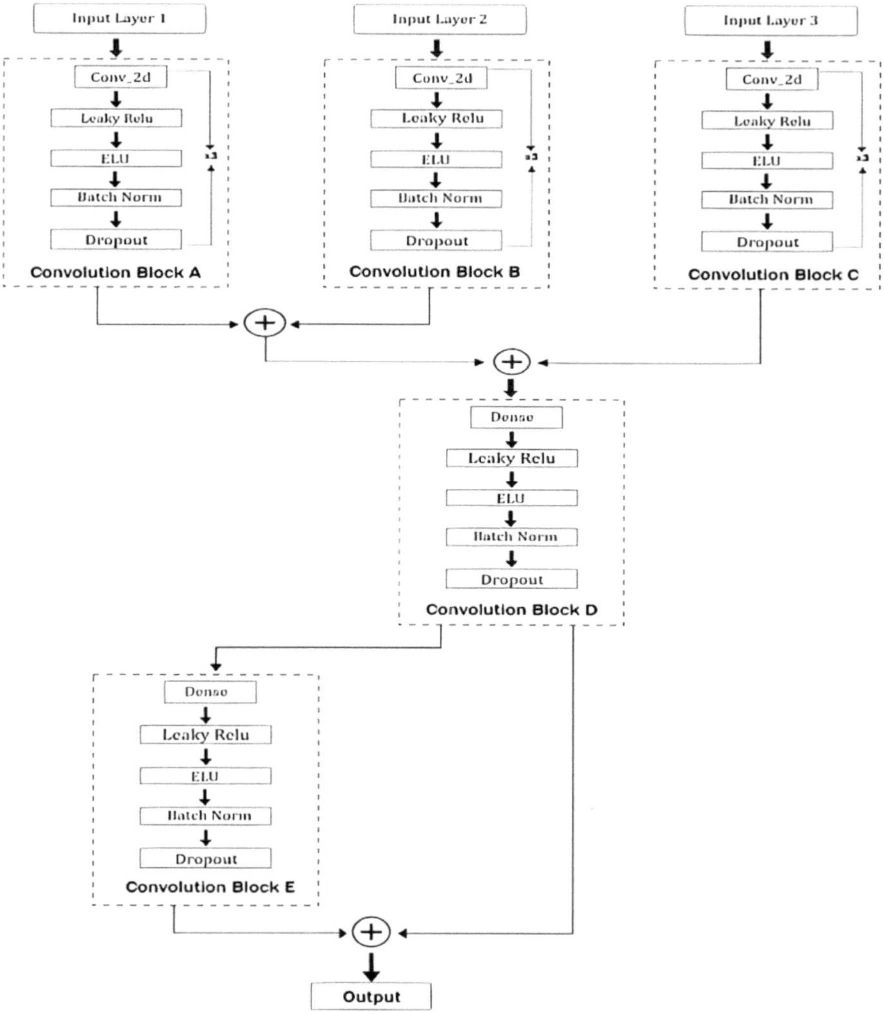

FIGURE 5.9 The block flow diagram of multimodal DCNN depicting the entire architectural details.

images it processed. The inputs to this Neural Network were initially reshaped into a 300x300x3 format, followed by a series of convolutional layers and max pooling operations. The design of the bimodal looping DCNN is reminiscent of residual networks, incorporating numerous skip connections for concatenating feature vectors from earlier stages, thus serving as our second component to support the Inception V3 network.

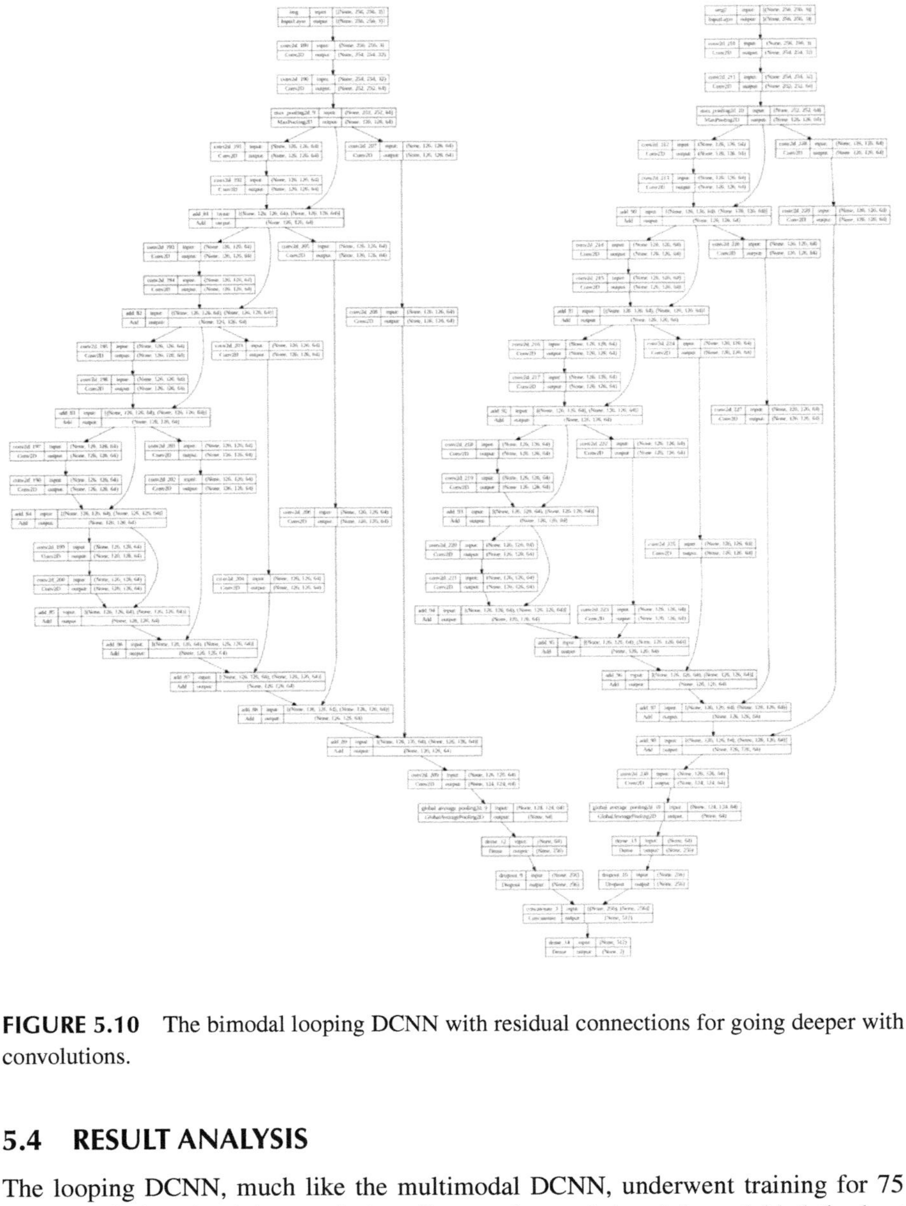

FIGURE 5.10 The bimodal looping DCNN with residual connections for going deeper with convolutions.

5.4 RESULT ANALYSIS

The looping DCNN, much like the multimodal DCNN, underwent training for 75 epochs utilizing the Adam optimizer. It was observed that Adam yielded the best results for this network when certain hyperparameters were carefully configured. The default learning rate was retained, while beta 1 and beta 2 were set to 0.87 and 0.888, respectively. Additionally, a fixed constant decay rate of 2.25e-08 with a slope of 2.25e-07 was applied. Notably, the training phase for this network was notably shorter than the previous one.

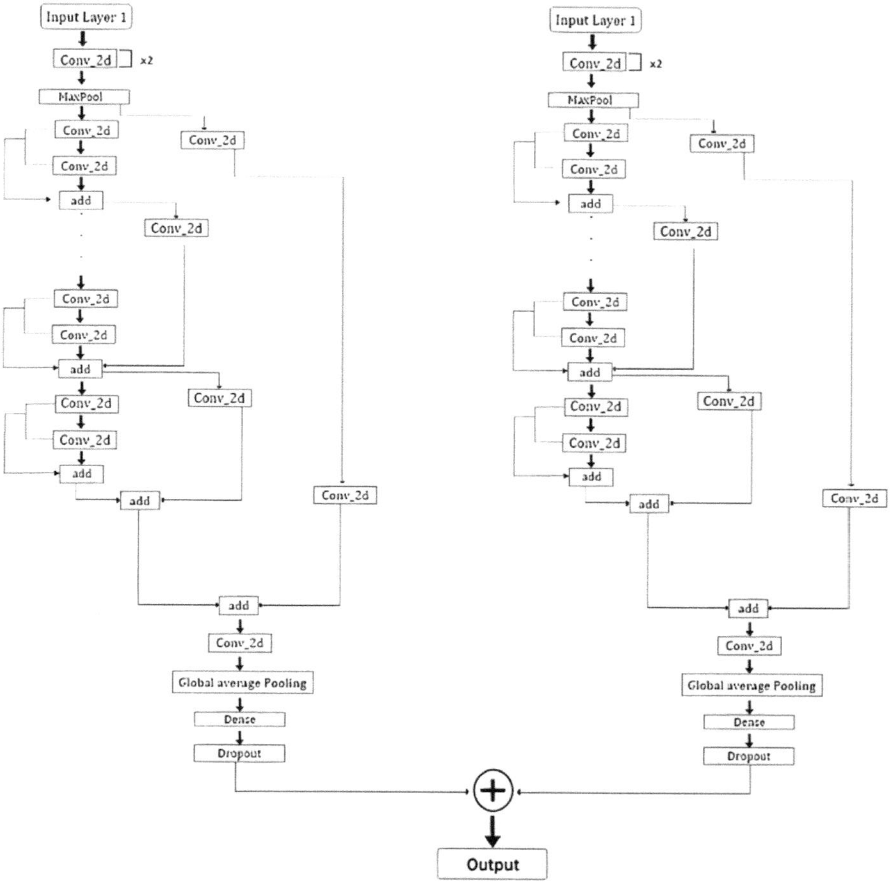

FIGURE 5.11 The block flow diagram of bimodal looping DCNN depicting the entire architectural details.

The looping DCNN boasted a total parameter count of 590,466, with all of these parameters being trainable. The design of the looping DCNN involved the nested application of convolution operations within inner layers. This approach allowed us to delve deeper into the network architecture while simultaneously reducing the overall number of parameters. It is worth mentioning that during training, there were moments when the proposed system exhibited a slight lag during validation. However, over time, the training and validation processes appeared to converge. Table 5.1 offers a more comprehensive overview of the multimodal DCNN for your reference.

Figure 5.12 shows the entire training performance of the multimodal DCNN. The model was able to achieve an accuracy of 98.49%, with a corresponding loss of 0.0373, as shown in Figure 5.12. While validation, the model was also able to perform quite well by achieving an accuracy of 91.92% and a corresponding loss of 0.5468. Thus, even from graph we can see that due to the absence of a good amount of data,

TABLE 5.1
Regarding the parameters of the multimodal DCNN

Layer Number	Layer Name	Layer Features	Layer Parameters	Additional Modifications	Default Values	Changed Values
1	Input Layer	Captures the inputs.	300x300x3	Three such layers for forming the convolutional feature extracting branch	Generally, 256x256x3 or 128x128x3 or 64x64x3	300x300x3
2	Convolutional Layer	32, 64 and 16 convolutional features for capturing details of the images	300x300x32, 300x300x64, and 300x300x16, respectively	One applied to each branch in a sequential manner for feature extraction.	Hyperparameter to tune around for better results.	150x150x32, 150x150x64, and 150x150x16, respectively.
3	Max pooling 2D layer	2x2 max pooling 2D layer to reduce feature map	150x150x32, 150x150x64, and 150x150x16, respectively, for three channels.	One applied to three branches in sequential manner.	2x2 is the default value of the pooling window with a stride of 1x1	2x2, and hence 75x75x64, 75x75x128 and 75x75x256 as the convolutions are applied.
4	Batch Normalization Layer	Applied to the inputs along axis of –1	150x150x32, 150x150x64, and 150x150x16, respectively, for three channels	Applied to each channel after a max pooling 2D layer for better training convergence	Default value of axis is -1, with momentum of 0.99 and epsilon of 1e-07	Axis kept at –1, with additional momentum of 0.85 and re-norm momentum of 0.97 with a change of epsilon of 2.25e-08

5	Leaky ReLU Activation Layer	Applied to outputs of the Batch Normalization Layer	150x150x32, 150x150x64, and 150x150x16, respectively	Applied to each layer after the max pooling 2D layer	Default value of alpha is 0.3	Value changed to 0.075 for better results during training error convergence.
6	Dropout Regularization Layer	Applied to outputs of the Leaky ReLU Activation Layer	150x150x32, 150x150x64, and 150x150x16, respectively, as before	Applied to each output of the Leaky ReLU Activation Layer again in a sequential format	Rate of dropout has no default value, decided on application designing	A dropout rate of 9% was kept constant for the convolutional layers.

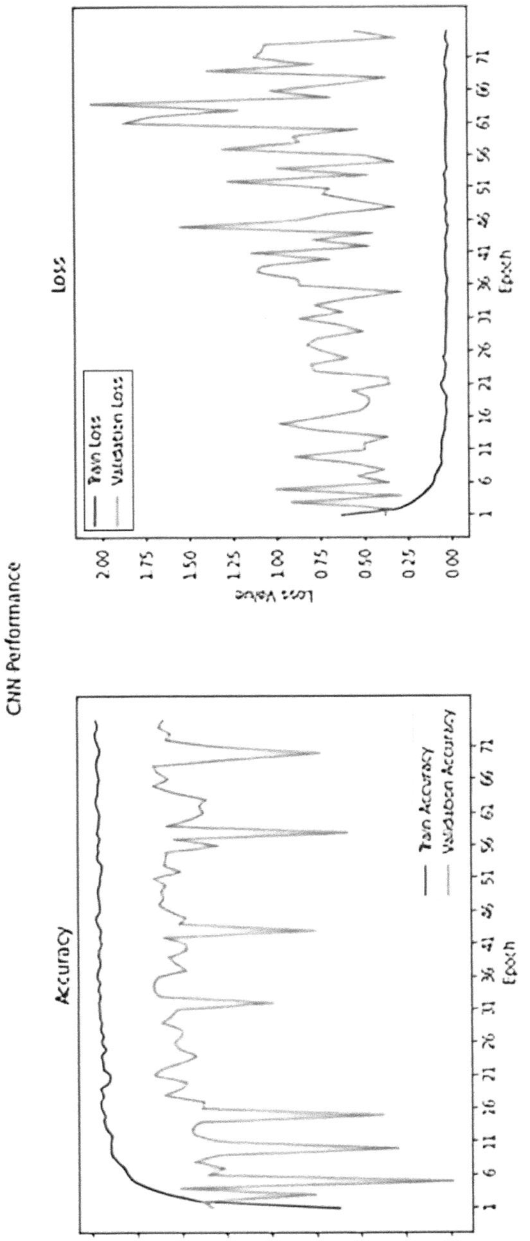

FIGURE 5.12 The performance graphs of the multimodal DCNN during training.

the model was unable to learn gradually, rather the learning was a bit abrupt and robust. CNNs tend to work very well while operating on images.

The principle of convolution is just matrix multiplication and replacing each value of the convolution matrix with the corresponding convoluted values. CNNs are always preferred over any other traditional deep learning or machine learning algorithms as the target can be easily achieved by a simple CNN as well as a complex logical CNN. Thus, while we were training the first component, it became very clear to us that the dataset is a bit tricky, so no naive or simple model can tackle with it. Deep learning always tends to be a bit more abstract as we cannot formulate such big notations in mathematics, which leads to the concept of black boxes solving some certain tasks.

The training accuracy seems to be a very impressive number as the multimodal DCNN was able to detect the malarial parasite images from the mixture of uninfected and parasitized images provided to it. The total number of parameters that the multimodal DCNN has is 57,081,576, with 57,079,010 trainable parameters and 2,496 non-trainable parameters. In any CNNs, we may find that the total number of trainable parameters is not exactly equal to the total parameters; rather there are some non-trainable parameters which are the contribution of the batch normalization layers, which we proposed to use in the three convolutional channels of the multimodal DCNN.

We trained the multimodal DCNN on an Nvidia Tesla P100, with a RAM of around 64 GB. The training was done on a small-scale data set due to time management. But surprisingly, our proposed CNN model, the multimodal DCNN, was an exception where people would say deep learning can't be applied on a small-scale image data set.

Figure 5.13 shows the performance graphs of the second component that will be acting like a support to the Inception V3, the Looping DCNN.

The training performance depicted in the figure above is undeniably impressive. During training, the looping DCNN achieved an accuracy of 98.25%, with a corresponding loss of 0.0175; while during validation, it reached a maximum accuracy of 97%, with a corresponding validation loss of 0.025. These performance graphs indicate that despite its depth and breadth, the looping DCNN was able to generalize well on testing samples, mitigating the risk of overfitting.

For optimizing the looping DCNN, we employed the Adam optimizer with specific hyperparameters. The learning rate was set to 0.00075, while beta_1 and beta_2 were held constant at 0.87 and 0.98, respectively. We opted for the Adam optimization algorithm because, unlike some other optimization techniques, it allowed the network to converge gradually, as evidenced by the performance graphs approaching their respective limits.

Here's a brief algorithmic description of the Adam (adaptive moments) optimizer with tuned hyperparameters, including beta_1, beta_2, a fixed decay of 2.25e-08, and epsilon set at 1.15e-07. The Adam optimizer was consistently chosen for all three CNNs: the looping DCNN, the multimodal DCNN, and the Inception V3 network. During training, each of these networks exceeded the 90% accuracy threshold and maintained an accuracy of over 85% during validation. The careful tuning of hyperparameters played a pivotal role in training these individual CNNs, ultimately resulting in their efficient generalization during the testing phase. In subsequent sections, we will delve into how the Adam optimization algorithm can be applied to CNN.

Figure 5.14 demonstrates how the performance graphs were for the Inception V3 network. In deep learning, the concept of transfer learning plays a vital role in

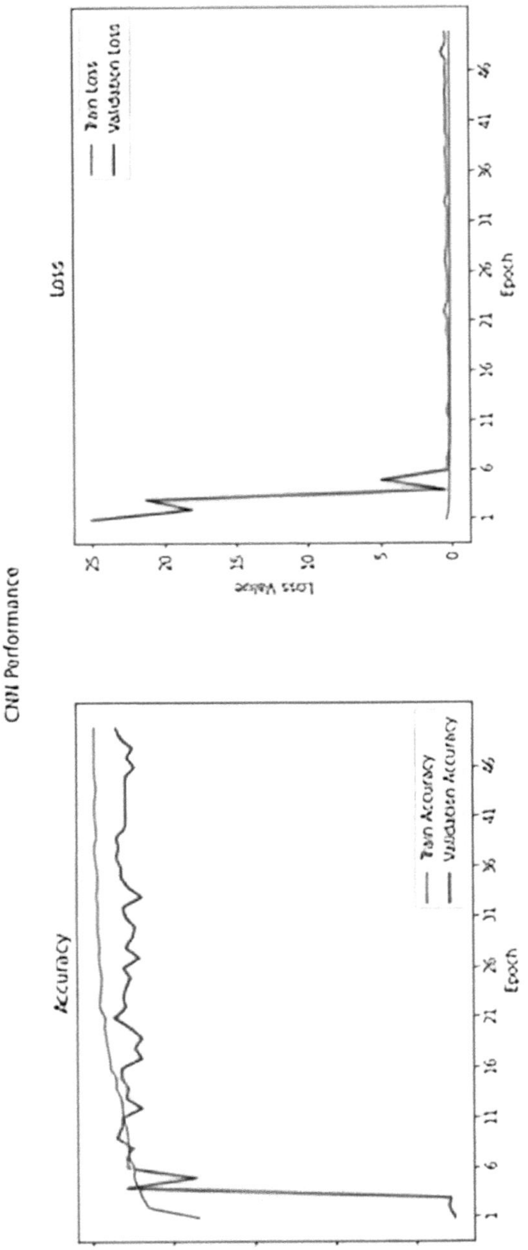

FIGURE 5.13 The performance graphs of the bimodal looping DCNN.

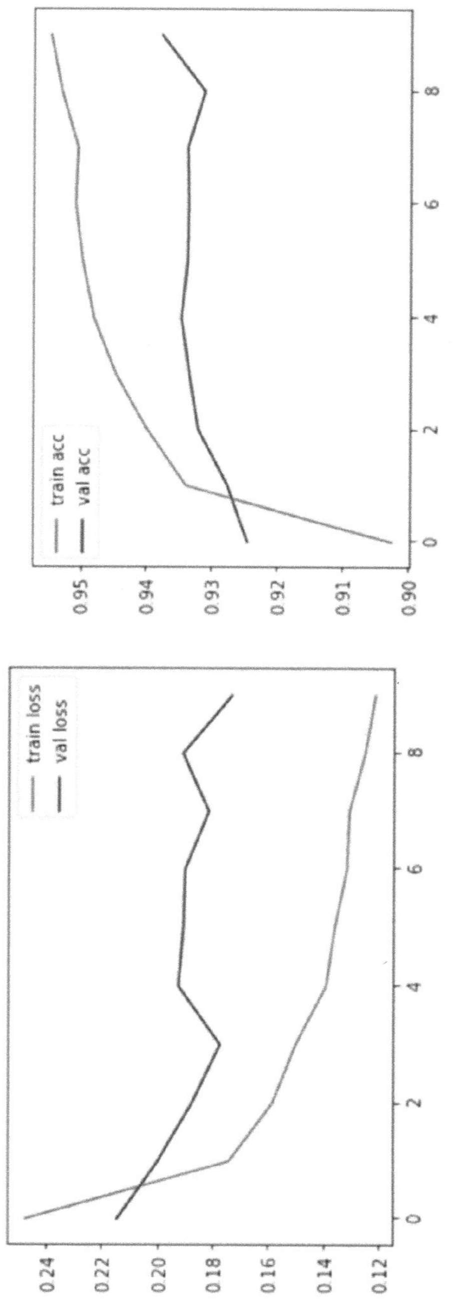

FIGURE 5.14 The performance graphs for the Inception V3 network.

TABLE 5.2
For the results obtained during training of the individual convolutional neural networks

Name of the Component	Optimizer Used	Optimizer Hyperparameters	Training Accuracy	Training Loss	Validation Accuracy	Validation Loss
The Multimodal Deep Convolutional Neural Network (DCNN)	Adaptive Moments Optimization (Adam optimizer)	Learning rate was 0.001, beta_1 was 0.87, beta_2 was 0.888, with decay and slope of 2.25e-08 and 2.25e-07, respectively.	98.49%	0.0373	91.92%	0.5468
The Bimodal Looping Deep Convolutional Neural Network (DCNN)	Adaptive Moments Optimization (Adam optimizer)	Learning rate was 0.00075, beta_1 and betal_2 were kept at 0.87 and 0.98, respectively, with a default value of decay and slope	98.25%	0.0175	97%	0.025
The Inception V3	Adam optimizer	Learning rate was 0.00085, beta_1 and betal_2 were kept at 0.75 and 0.85, respectively, with a default value of epsilon and decay was kept at 1.75e-08	98%	0.054	97.25%	0.0757

solving real-world problems. The Inception V3 network proposed by Google was open sourced in 2014 via Python upon TensorFlow and PyTorch. In this work, we have used the Inception V3 network for the detection of malarial parasite from cell images.

The network itself is quite complicated for us to formulate. In earlier sections, details regarding the components of Inception V3 were explained. Google proposed this network in their paper coined as "Going Deeper with Convolutions," which overshoot the current state-of-the-art algorithms. Inception V3 was trained on the ImageNet dataset. The dataset itself is quite huge consisting of high-resolution images of around 1,000 different categories.

The state-of-the-art results were quite robust for the Inception V3 network and hence it replaced the existing state of the art. The Inception V3 network was used in the work via transfer learning. The network is comprised of around 224 layers and the main idea behind the working is the dimensional reduction of images in consequent steps as well as going deep with convolutions. Regarding the training of the Inception V3 network, we proposed to train it with the minimum number of epochs possible as wanted to train the network from scratch. The training of the Inception V3 was done for the least time, around 35 epochs with conditional decaying learning rate scheduler and early stopping. The obtained results were not only robust but also converging to the thresholds of accuracy and loss.

The Inception V3 network was trained for around 35 epochs but within 15 epochs, the early stopping was applied and thus the model's training phase was over with a training accuracy of 98% and a training loss of 0.054, while validation accuracy seems to be saturated at around 97.25%, with a corresponding validation loss of 0.0757. Thus, the obtained results were quite awesome for the system to detect the presence of any malarial parasite. Once again the entire training of the ensemble system was done in a heavy work station with a RAM of 64GB and a GPU of Nvidia Tesla P100 having 16 GB of memory. For further training, the time consumption can't be minimized due to extensive resource usage. The final obtained results are also provided in a tabular format in the next sections. Learning rate for the Inception V3 training was kept fixed at 0.00085, with beta_1 and beta_2 at 0.75 and 0.85, respectively, along with a decay value of 1.75e-08 and epsilon fixed at a default value (Table 5.2).

5.5 DISCUSSION

From Table 5.2 we can clearly conclude that each of the neural networks was able to generalize upon the validation data and also the metrics were quite outstanding. Using these three CNNs in an ensemble way like bagging can be very much useful for more accurate prediction as we must be cautioned enough to deal with medical data. The three CNNs were able to justify the dataset by properly detecting the presence of any malarial parasite. Deep learning allows us to create many robust and advanced architecture that can solve many detection and classification tasks. Creating an ensemble system of many neural networks can be of great advantage. The ensemble learning system is way more accurate and robust than any single neural network. Thus, our proposed systems of three CNNs are capable enough to deal with the malarial parasite detection problem and were able to justify it as well. Figure 5.14 demonstrates the learned features of the ensemble system during combined predictions. CNNs are great in learning different image features, and thus predicting accordingly matching with the learned features. The features that the CNNs learn while training are the main criteria of selecting whether a malarial parasite is present or not; if certain features are matched with certain image inputs, then the detection is done perfectly. CNNs are thus, very much useful while dealing with images of different categories (Figure 5.15).

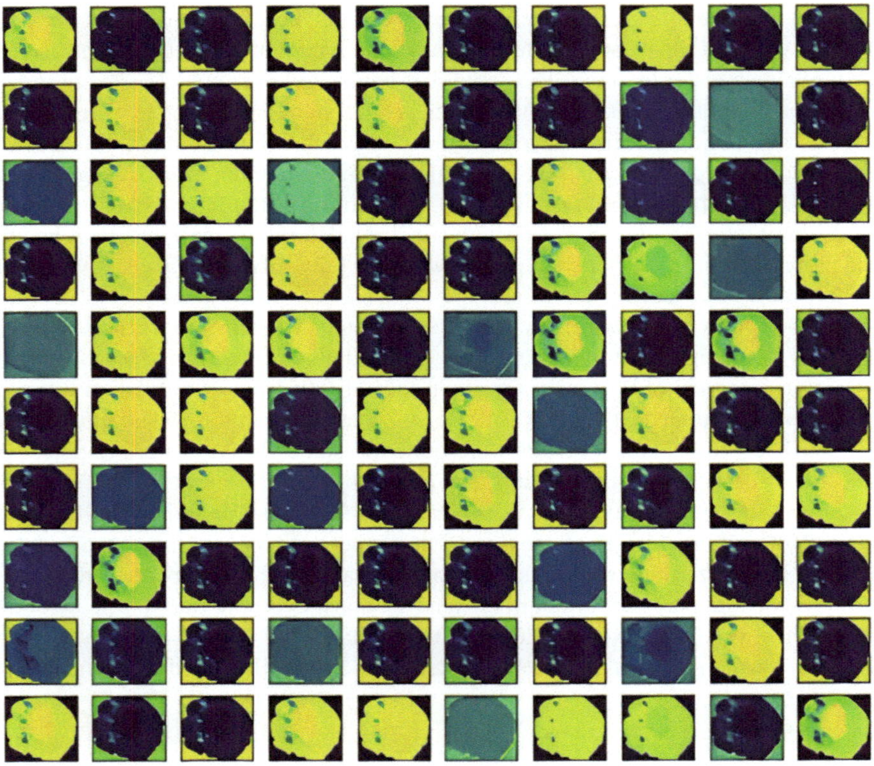

FIGURE 5.15 The features learned from different malarial images.

Along with the features of the malarial parasite images, we have also provided the features that were captured during the analysis of the images that were not infected by malarial parasite. These features are the guiding factor for the justification of whether an image of cell is affected by the malarial parasite or not. Thus, we have provided the feature map in Figure 5.16.

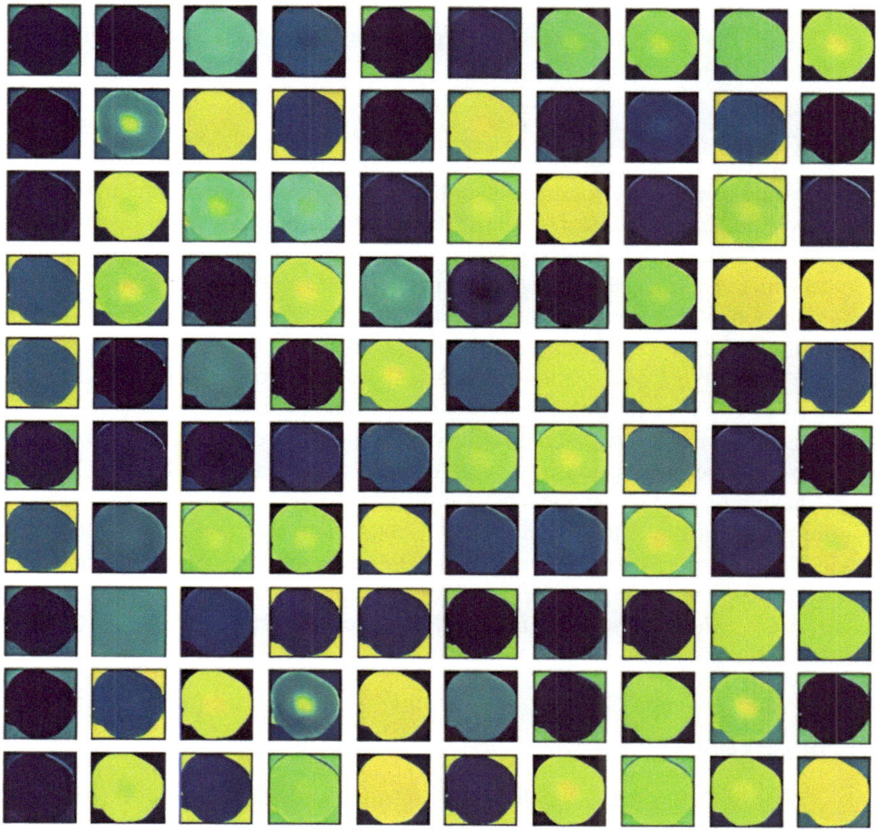

FIGURE 5.16 The features learned from different non-malarial images.

CNNs are thus very useful when we deal with high-quality images. Some applications of CNNs are also provided below.

Applications of CNN image classification:

- Image classification is the task of classifying an image into one of a set of classes. For example, given an image, classify it as an image of a cat or, say, a dog.
- Image recognition is the task of identifying objects or their instances in an image. For example, given an image, identify and count the number of cats in the image.
- Object detection is the task of finding the location and the type of objects present in an image. For example, given an image, detect if there is a door present in the image and the location where it is present, etc.

- Semantic segmentation is the task of classifying pixels in an image into different classes. For example, given an image, separate the background from objects present in the image.

5.6 CONCLUSION

Deep learning can be very robust and sophisticated while dealing with large amount of quality data. In this chapter we have demonstrated how a type of deep learning algorithm coined as CNN can be applied on high-quality images to justify the category to which that image belongs. Neural networks are always used in the field of big data and exponentially growing data. In this work we have used such CNNs together for training and also creating an ensemble learning system of the former so as to deal with the problem of detection of malarial parasite beforehand just by supplying images of both parasitized and uninfected cells. The proposed system was able to tackle the problem as we have created the ensemble system. Once again it was found that CNNs can be very handy in case of dealing with images. But the architecture that we have proposed was made a bit complicated so as to ensure better detection of malarial parasite from some given inputs of both uninfected and parasitized images of cells. In medical research and technology, this detection of malarial parasite in an automated way can be of great help and also the time for the real-time detection of the parasite is reduced as we have now a CNN system that can deal with the detection of malarial cell parasites.

REFERENCES

1. Szegedy, C., Liu, W., Jia, Y., Sermanet, P., Reed, S., Anguelov, D., Erhan, D., Vanhoucke, V. and Rabinovich, A., 2015. Going deeper with convolutions. In *Proceedings of the IEEE conference on computer vision and pattern recognition.*
2. Shen, D., Wu, G. and Suk, H.I., 2017. Deep learning in medical image analysis. *Annual Review of Biomedical Engineering*, 19, pp. 221–248.
3. Suzuki, K., 2017. Overview of deep learning in medical imaging. *Radiological Physics and Technology*, 10(3), pp. 257–273.
4. Razzak, M.I., Naz, S. and Zaib, A., 2018. Deep learning for medical image processing: Overview, challenges and the future. *Classification in BioApps*, pp. 323–350.
5. Chang, J., Yu, J., Han, T., Chang, H.J. and Park, E., 2017, October. A method for classifying medical images using transfer learning: A pilot study on histopathology of breast cancer. In *2017 IEEE 19th international conference on e-health networking, applications and services (Healthcom)* (pp. 1–4). IEEE.
6. Saini, M. and Susan, S., 2019, July. Data augmentation of minority class with transfer learning for classification of imbalanced breast cancer dataset using inception-V3. In *Iberian conference on pattern recognition and image analysis* (pp. 409–420). Springer, Cham.
7. Zhou, S., Zhang, X. and Zhang, R., 2019. Identifying cardiomegaly in ChestX-ray8 using transfer learning. In *MEDINFO 2019: Health and Wellbeing e-Networks for All* (pp. 482–486). IOS Press.
8. Wang, C., Chen, D., Hao, L., Liu, X., Zeng, Y., Chen, J. and Zhang, G., 2019. Pulmonary image classification based on inception-v3 transfer learning model. *IEEE Access*, 7, pp. 146533–146541.

9. Dong, N., Zhao, L., Wu, C.H. and Chang, J.F., 2020. Inception v3 based cervical cell classification combined with artificially extracted features. *Applied Soft Computing*, 93, p. 106311.
10. Mednikov, Y., Nehemia, S., Zheng, B., Benzaquen, O. and Lederman, D., 2018, July. Transfer representation learning using Inception-V3 for the detection of masses in mammography. In *2018 40th Annual international conference of the IEEE Engineering in Medicine and Biology Society (EMBC)* (pp. 2587–2590).
11. Yadav, S.S. and Jadhav, S.M., 2019. Deep convolutional neural network based medical image classification for disease diagnosis. *Journal of Big Data*, 6(1), pp. 1–18.
12. Xie, Y. and Richmond, D., 2018. Pre-training on grayscale imagenet improves medical image classification. In *Proceedings of the European conference on computer vision (ECCV) workshops*.
13. Hsieh, Y.C., Chin, C.L., Wei, C.S., Chen, I.M., Yeh, P.Y. and Tseng, R.J., 2020, November. Combining VGG16, Mask R-CNN and Inception V3 to identify the benign and malignant of breast microcalcification clusters. In *2020 International conference on fuzzy theory and its applications (iFUZZY)* (pp. 1–4).
14. Ramaneswaran, S., Srinivasan, K., Vincent, P.M. and Chang, C.Y., 2021. Hybrid Inception v3 XGBoost model for acute lymphoblastic leukemia classification. *Computational and Mathematical Methods in Medicine* .
15. Pelka, O., Nensa, F. and Friedrich, C.M., 2018. Annotation of enhanced radiographs for medical image retrieval with deep convolutional neural networks. *PloS One*, 13(11), p. e0206229.
16. Liu, Z., Yang, C., Huang, J., Liu, S., Zhuo, Y. and Lu, X., 2021. Deep learning framework based on integration of S-Mask R-CNN and Inception-v3 for ultrasound image-aided diagnosis of prostate cancer. *Future Generation Computer Systems*, 114, pp. 358–367.
17. Li, J., Wang, P., Li, Y., Zhou, Y., Liu, X. and Luan, K., 2018, August. Transfer learning of pre-trained inception-V3 model for colorectal cancer lymph node metastasis classification. In *2018 IEEE international conference on mechatronics and automation (ICMA)* (pp. 1650–1654).
18. Gaur, L., Bhatia, U., Jhanjhi, N.Z., Muhammad, G. and Masud, M., 2021. Medical image-based detection of COVID-19 using deep convolution neural networks. *Multimedia Systems*.
19. Graziani, M., Lompech, T., Müller, H., Depeursinge, A. and Andrearczyk, V., 2020. Interpretable CNN pruning for preserving scale-covariant features in medical imaging. In *Interpretable and Annotation-Efficient Learning for Medical Image Computing* (pp. 23–32). Cham: Springer.
20. Khan, H.A., Jue, W., Mushtaq, M. and Mushtaq, M.U., 2020. Brain tumor classification in MRI image using convolutional neural network.
21. Kim, J.Y. and Ye, S.Y., 2019. Accuracy evaluation of brain parenchymal MRI image classification using Inception V3. *Journal of the Institute of Convergence Signal Processing*, 20(3), pp. 132–137.
22. Wang, S., Shi, J., Ye, Z., Dong, D., Yu, D., Zhou, M., Liu, Y., Gevaert, O., Wang, K., Zhu, Y. and Zhou, H., 2019. Predicting EGFR mutation status in lung adenocarcinoma on computed tomography image using deep learning. *European Respiratory Journal*.
23. Lee, T.Y., Huang, K.Y., Chuang, C.H., Lee, C.Y. and Chang, T.H., 2020. Incorporating deep learning and multi-omics autoencoding for analysis of lung adenocarcinoma prognostication. *Computational Biology and Chemistry*, 87, p. 107277.

24. Zhao, W., Zhang, W., Sun, Y., Ye, Y., Yang, J., Chen, W., Gao, P., Li, J., Li, C., Jin, L. and Wang, P., 2019. Convolution kernel and iterative reconstruction affect the diagnostic performance of radiomics and deep learning in lung adenocarcinoma pathological subtypes. *Thoracic Cancer*, 10(10), pp. 1893–1903.
25. Alsubaie, N., Shaban, M., Snead, D., Khurram, A. and Rajpoot, N., 2018, July. A multi-resolution deep learning framework for lung adenocarcinoma growth pattern classification. In *Annual conference on medical image understanding and analysis* (pp. 3–11). Cham: Springer.
26. Wang, J., Xie, X., Shi, J., He, W., Chen, Q., Chen, L., Gu, W. and Zhou, T., 2020. Denoising Autoencoder, a deep learning algorithm, aids the identification of a novel molecular signature of lung adenocarcinoma. *Genomics, Proteomics & Bioinformatics*.
27. Yanagawa, M., Niioka, H., Hata, A., Kikuchi, N., Honda, O., Kurakami, H., Morii, E., Noguchi, M., Watanabe, Y., Miyake, J. and Tomiyama, N., 2019. Application of deep learning (3-dimensional convolutional neural network) for the prediction of pathological invasiveness in lung adenocarcinoma: A preliminary study. *Medicine*, 98(25).
28. Tsirikoglou, A., Stacke, K., Eilertsen, G., Lindvall, M. and Unger, J., 2020. A study of deep learning colon cancer detection in limited data access scenarios. *arXiv preprint arXiv:2005.10326*.

6 Implementation of a Deep Convolutional Auto-Encoding Image-Reconstruction Network (DCARN) to Visualize Distinct Categories of COVID-19 and Pneumonia X-Ray Image Features

6.1 INTRODUCTION

Convolutional neural networks (CNNs) have been used extensively in deep learning up to this point. For further information, see Chapters 2, 3, and 4. These deep learning CNN methods outperform other conventional machine learning techniques for image identification tasks like demonstrated in [1, 2 and 3]. However, the underlying idea frequently remains a mystery. In this chapter, a method for fully comprehending the operation of CNN is suggested. This method uses a deep convolutional auto-encoder architecture (Figure 6.1).

Auto-encodes have numerous uses in the fields of deep learning and image processing. In the past, we have observed how well our artificial intelligence (AI) systems for image recognition of COVID-19 X-ray pictures of the lungs and, later, for the detection of categories of pneumonia, also using X-ray images, tend to work. Both Chapters 4 and 5 concentrated on how systems were implemented using CNNs and transfer learning, but neither chapter really outlined why certain architectures typically perform so well. The auto-encoder diagram for the application of image reconstruction on the MNIST dataset is shown in Figure 6.1. The idea of probability distributions serves as the foundation for auto-encoders (AEs). The AE attempts to learn the probability distribution of the inputs, (X), during the training process so that

DOI: 10.1201/9781003456476-6

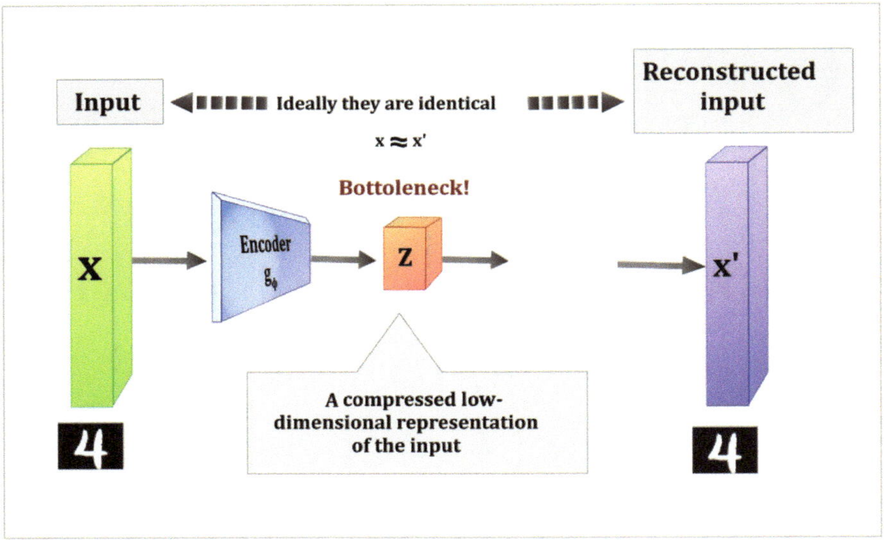

FIGURE 6.1 The auto-encoder architecture for the application of domain-specific image reconstruction. (The generation of same inputs from the MNIST dataset.)

subsequently it is able to create the outputs, (X), as well. The primary goal of AEs is the idea of linear pixel matching. The major object of concern is the equation.

$$\text{Input distribution} = \text{Output distribution}$$
$$X = X'$$

The encoder network and the decoder network are two domain-specific neural networks that make up the auto-encoder architecture. The job of the encoder is to turn each input into a corresponding encoded vector matrix, which is then supplied to the decoder for a final transformation back into the original shape of each input. In order to grasp the hidden underlying features that are present in the inputs, the encoder changes the input to the encoded space during training, and the decoder attempts to convert the encoded space to the shape of the input.

6.2 THE AUTO-ENCODER ARCHITECTURE

A unique kind of neural network called auto-encoder is taught to replicate its input in its output. For instance, an auto-encoder will encode a handwritten digit image into a lower dimensional latent representation, then decode the latent representation back into the original image. A strong technique for dimensionality reduction, an auto-encoder learns to compress the data while minimizing the reconstruction error. The AEs' basic operating principle is the production of probability distributions from an input probability distribution. AEs come in a wide variety of forms, but they all have a similar fundamental structure. Figure 6.2 shows an auto-encoder made up of an artificial neural network serving as both the encoder and the decoder. This kind of architecture, which essentially consists of many inputs and multiple output neural networks, can produce data sequences that are independent of time.

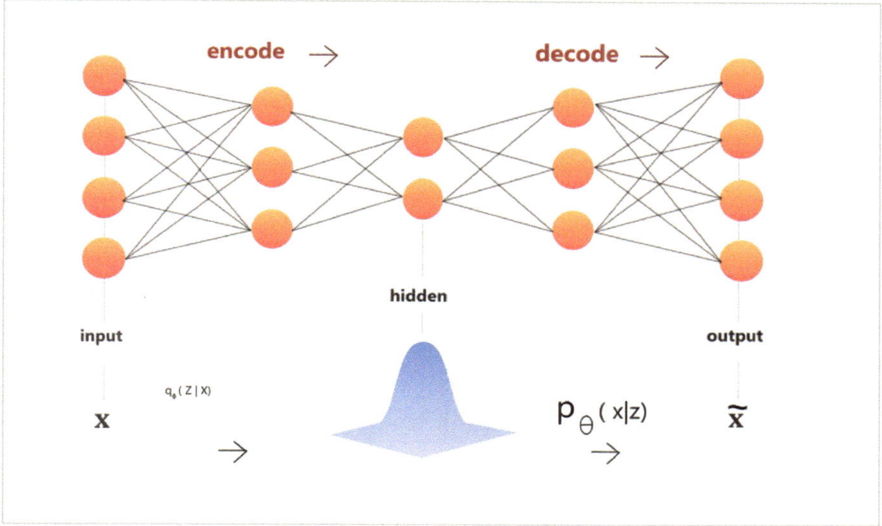

FIGURE 6.2 The auto-encoder comprising input, hidden, and output layers.

An auto-encoder has three layers:

- An input layer
- A hidden layer
- An output layer.

The data is introduced into the system at the input layer, compressed at the hidden layer, and decoded at the output layer. The number of neurons in the input layer and the number of neurons in the hidden layer are two crucial variables that affect how an auto-encoder functions. How much data is fed into the auto-encoder depends on how many neurons are present in the input layer. The amount of information compressed depends on how many neurons are present in the buried layer. Data will be compressed more by an auto-encoder with fewer hidden layer neurons than by an auto-encoder with more hidden layer neurons. This is due to the fact that fewer neurons in the hidden layer will learn to accurately represent the data than more neurons will, providing the deeper layer more power to recognize and capture better hidden features. Domain adaptation, picture reconstruction, anomaly detection, image denoising, and many other uses are a few of the applications of AEs. The architecture of the encoder and decoder determines the type of auto-encoder. Simple auto-encoding refers to an encoder with no hidden layers, whereas convolutional auto-encoding uses convolutional networks as the encoder. The encoder used in anomaly detection is often a Long Short Term Memory Recurrent Neural Network (LSTM-RNN) network.

6.2.1 Convolutional Auto-Encoder

Convolutional auto-encoders (CAEs), a subtype of CNNs, are employed for unsupervised learning of convolution filters. Typically, they find applications in image reconstruction tasks with the aim of minimizing reconstruction errors by discovering optimal filters. Once trained for this purpose, they can extract features from various inputs [4, 5]. In contrast to traditional AEs, which do not consider the inherent 2D structure of images, CAEs serve as versatile feature extractors. However, AEs require the input image to be flattened into a single vector, and the network architecture must be designed with scalability in mind to handle a multitude of inputs. CAEs utilize a set of learned filters to perform convolutions on input images, thereby acquiring a compact representation of the input data. A convolutional auto-encoder is constructed by incorporating a stack of convolutional layers into a multi-layered auto-encoder, which is then fully connected. This architecture comprises a series of convolutional layers followed by a fully connected layer to create a complete convolutional auto-encoder. These models can be used to solve any medical problem as well like that mentioned in [6 and 7].

Figure 6.3 shows the architecture of a three-layer convolutional auto-encoder.

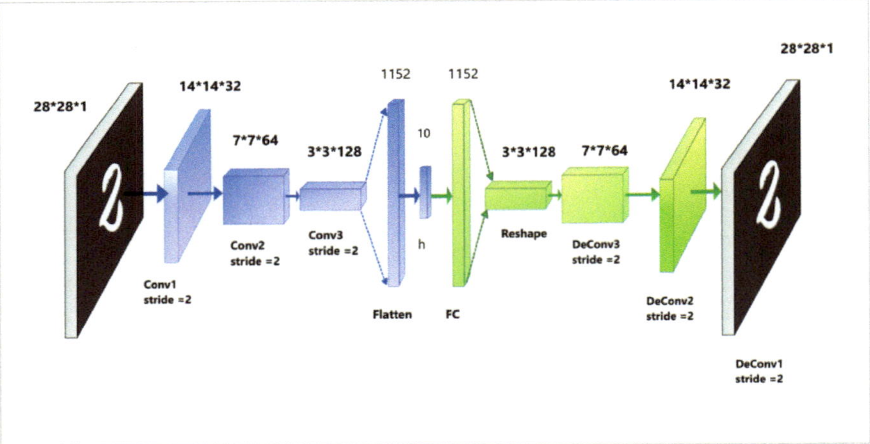

FIGURE 6.3 Convolutional auto-encoder neural network.

The convolutional auto-encoder architecture follows a specific flow. It begins with an input that is processed through a series of convolutional layers, each followed by a fully connected layer. The final outcome of this series is a compressed representation of the input, which is the output of the last fully connected layer. The complete structure of the convolutional auto-encoder, designed for reconstructing domain-specific images from the MNIST dataset, is illustrated in Figure 6.3.

Within the context of the MNIST dataset, the primary aim of the convolutional auto-encoder is to generate handwritten digit images based on provided inputs. The resulting generated images serve as reconstructions of the input images. Figure 6.3 presents an illustration of how convolutional layers transform the inputs into a latent space vector [8, 9 and 10], while the transpose convolutional decoder works to convert this encoded vector back into generated images corresponding to the original inputs. The decoder component plays a central role in this process, striving to reconstruct the input image from the compressed representation created by the encoder [11 and 12].

To elucidate this concept, consider an example: Suppose we commence with an input image measuring 28×28 pixels. Traditionally, this image is flattened, resulting in a (784)-pixel representation before feeding it into the neural network. The encoder block, the initial segment of the network, takes this representation as input. The output of the encoder is then directed to the bottleneck, also referred to as the latent space, where it undergoes a reduction in dimensionality. For instance, if we choose to have 8, 16, or any number of nodes in the latent space, it implies that we have effectively compressed an image originally composed of 784 pixels down to only 8 nodes, 16 nodes, or the chosen number of nodes.

The decoder network then undertakes the task of reconstructing the original (28×28) input image from this compressed state within the bottleneck. The operation proceeds as follows: After the image has been successfully reconstructed, a comparison is drawn between the reconstructed image and the original image. The discrepancy between these two images is calculated, resulting in the computation of a loss function that quantifies their dissimilarity. The overarching objective is to minimize this loss function, which essentially guides the network in the process of learning to generate accurate reconstructions.

The loss is calculated by:

$$L(\theta, \varphi) = \frac{1}{n} \Sigma_{i=1}^{n} \left(x^i - f_\theta \left(g_\varphi \left(x^i \right) \right) \right)^2$$

6.2.2 The Mathematical Modeling of a Convolutional Auto-Encoder

The convolution operator plays a critical role in signal processing, allowing for the extraction of specific features from an input signal. However, traditional AEs do not typically consider the idea that a signal could be represented as a sum of various other signals.

In contrast, CAEs leverage this concept by employing the convolution operator. These AEs aim to reconstruct the input signal by learning to encode it into a set of simpler signals. In essence, they learn to represent the input as a combination of these simpler signals, which can lead to more effective feature extraction and reconstruction.

Since a convolution is defined as the integral of the product of two functions (signals) in the general case after one of them has been shifted and reversed, the convolution operation can be explained using the integral form of mathematics and thus can be demonstrated as: $f(t) * g(t) =^{def} \int_{-\infty}^{\infty} f(\tau) g(t-\tau) d\tau$

Consequently, a convolution results in a new function (signal). Considering that the convolution is a commutative operation, we can formulate like $f(t)*g(t)=g(t)*f(t)$.

In a general n-dimensional space, AEs may be taught to decode (encode(x)) inputs for the purpose of reconstructing images. AEs are frequently employed in the real world to extract features from 2D, discrete, and finite input signals, such as digital photographs.

In the 2D discrete space, the convolution operation is defined as:

$$O(i,j)=\sum_{u=-\infty}^{\infty}\sum_{v=-\infty}^{\infty}F(u,v)I(i-u,j-v)$$

CAEs introduce an innovative approach to filter development. Instead of manually designing convolutional filters, CAEs enable the model to autonomously discover the most effective filters by minimizing the reconstruction error. Once these filters have been trained, they can be applied to various computer vision tasks. Modern tools for unsupervised learning, such as CAEs, make it possible to extract features from any input data. These learned features can then be utilized in a wide range of tasks that require a compact representation of the input, including classification and other computer vision applications.

CAEs are a type of CNN: The key distinction between CNNs and CAEs, as commonly understood, lies in their training objectives and approaches. CNNs are typically trained end-to-end for tasks like filter learning and feature integration, primarily aimed at classifying input data. These networks often use supervised learning methods. On the other hand, CAEs are specifically trained to learn filters that can efficiently extract features capable of reconstructing the input data. CAEs prioritize feature extraction for reconstruction rather than classification. Due to their convolutional architecture, CAEs exhibit scalability to handle large high-dimensional images while maintaining a constant number of parameters for building activation maps. In contrast, traditional AEs do not consider the 2D structure of images. AEs require a fixed number of inputs and demand the image to be flattened into a single vector, constraining their applicability compared to the more versatile CAEs.

6.2.3 The Convolutional Encoder of the CAEs

The fact that a single convolutional filter cannot learn to extract the wide variety of patterns that make up an image is simple to comprehend. Due to this, each convolutional layer is made up of n (hyperparameter) convolutional filters with a depth of D, where D is the depth of the input. Therefore, a convolution among an input volume $I=\{I_1,\cdots,I_D\}$ and a set of n convolutional filters $\{F_1^{(1)},\cdots,F_n^{(1)}\}$, each with depth D, produces a set of n activation maps, or equivalently, a volume of activation maps with depth n:

$$O_m(i,j)=a\left(\sum_{d=1}^{D}\sum_{u=-2k-1}^{2k+1}\sum_{v=-2k-1}^{2k+1}F_{m_d}^{(1)}(u,v)I_d(i-u,j-v)\right)$$

$$m = 1,\cdots,n$$

To improve the generalization capabilities of the network, every convolution is wrapped by a non-linear function a (activation); in that way the training procedure can learn to represent input combining non-linear functions:

$$z_m = O_m = a\left(I * F_m^{(1)} + b_m^{(1)}\right) m = 1,\cdots,m$$

where $b_m^{(1)}$ is the bias (single real value for every activation map) for the mth feature map. To use the same variable name as the latent variable used in the AEs, the term z_m has been introduced. The generated activation maps represent the encoding of the input I in a low-dimensional space, where "low-dimensional" refers to the number of parameters required to construct each feature map rather than the width and height of O, O_m, or the quantity of parameters to be learned. We need a decoding process with the ability to rebuild the input I from the generated feature maps because that is what we want to achieve. Since CAEs are entirely convolutional networks, the decoding process also involves convolutions.

6.2.4 The Convolutional Decoder of the CAEs

The produced n feature maps $z_{m=1,\cdots,n}$ (latent representations) will be used as input to the decoder in order to reconstruct the input image I from this reduced representation. The hyperparameters of the decoding convolution are fixed by the encoding architecture, for filters volume $F^{(2)}$ with dimensions$(2k+1, 2k+1, n)$, because the convolution should span across every feature map and produce a volume with the same spatial extent of I. The number of filters to learn: D, because we're interested in reconstructing the input image that has depth D. Therefore, the reconstructed image $I^{\sim}$ is the result of the convolution between the volume of feature maps $Z = \left\{z_{i=1}\right\}^n$ and this convolutional filter volume $F^{(2)}$. Thus, we can say that $I^{\sim} = a\left(Z * F_m^{(2)} + b^{(2)}\right)$.

Padding I with the previously found number of zeros leads the decoding convolution to produce a volume with dimensions: $O_w = O_h = \left(I_w + (2k+1) - 1\right) - (2k+1) + 1 = I_w = I_h$.

Having input's dimensions equal to the output's dimensions, it is possible to relate input and output using any loss function, like the MSE:

$$L\left(I, I^{\sim}\right) = \frac{1}{2} \| I - I^{\sim} \|_2^2$$

The primary objective of the auto-primary encoder is to minimize the loss function specific to the associated domain application. Another type of AE that can be developed to address this issue is the variational auto-encoder (VAE). VAEs operate on similar principles as AEs but introduce modifications to the encoded latent space produced by the encoder.

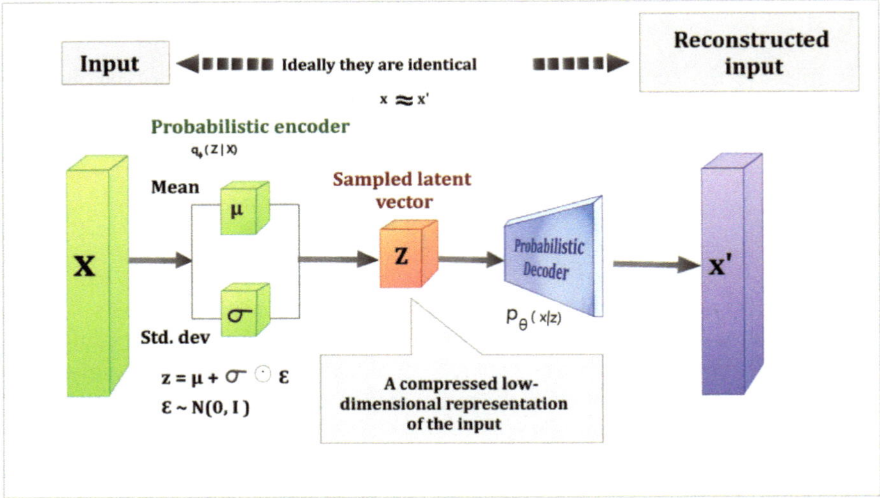

FIGURE 6.4 Reconstructed input generation methodology.

Figure 6.4 illustrates the architecture of the VAE. In the figure, we can observe that the structure of the VAE's encoder is similar to that of a traditional AE, except for a change in the penultimate stage of the encoder. The latent space vector generated by the encoder's output is determined by the mean and standard deviation of the penultimate output of the encoder. These mean and standard deviation values, along with the involvement of probability distributions, govern the generation of encoded data. The central component of the VAE lies in the division of the encoder's mean and standard deviation.

In general, AEs and VAEs share many similarities. The key distinction between them is that the bottleneck of the VAE is continuous and consists of two separate vectors: one representing the means of the distribution and the other representing the standard deviations of the distribution. Since the loss function in an AE is simple and compact and does not involve mean and standard deviation components, optimizing the loss function is relatively straightforward. The loss function minimized by the AE during training is expressed below.

Auto-encoder loss function: $-L(\theta,\varphi)=\frac{1}{n}\sum_{i=1}^{n}\left(x^i-f_\theta\left(g_\varphi\left(x^i\right)\right)\right)^2$ (referred earlier)

Variational auto-encoder loss function: $L(\theta,\varphi)=-E_{z\sim q_\theta}\left[P_\theta(x\mid z)\right]+D_{KL}\left(q_\varphi(z\mid x)\parallel p_\theta(z)\right)$

As we can see, the loss function of the VAE differs slightly from that of the AE. The reconstruction loss and the regularizer, which is essentially a Kullback–Leibler Divergence between the encoder's distribution and the latent space, define the VAE loss function. The operation of the VAE is illustrated in Figure 6.5.

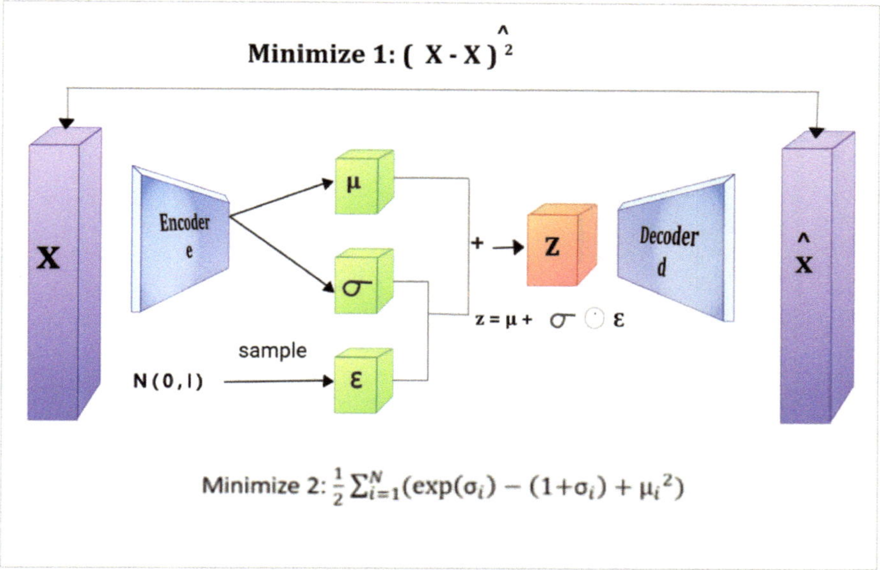

FIGURE 6.5 The working of a variational auto-encoder for image reconstruction.

VAEs are a type of AE that utilizes a variational approach to learn the latent space of data. In VAEs, the encoder is a probabilistic model responsible for mapping input data to a latent space, while the decoder maps the latent space back to the original input data. By optimizing a lower bound on the log-likelihood of the data, the variational approach allows VAEs to acquire a more accurate representation of the data.

VAEs excel at learning precise data representations because they can leverage the latent space to capture a richer set of data information compared to a standard AE. These models have demonstrated their effectiveness in learning complex data representations and have been applied to enhance the performance of various machine learning algorithms.

6.3 IMPLEMENTATION OF THE PROPOSED DCARN (AKA DEEP CONVOLUTIONAL AUTO-ENCODING IMAGE RECONSTRUCTION NETWORK)

As demonstrated earlier, AEs have the capability to reconstruct images within a given domain. In our work, we have applied this concept to the reconstruction of four different types of X-ray images. These include the reconstruction of X-ray images from COVID-19 pneumonia patients, non-COVID-19 lung infection X-ray images, normal lung X-ray images, and viral-pneumonia X-ray images. The dataset used for training the AE consists of the datasets we employed in Chapters 3 and 4 of this book. Chapter 3 focused on proposing an advanced method for detecting COVID-19 from chest X-ray images, while Chapter 4 aimed to detect pneumonia variants using lung X-rays once again.

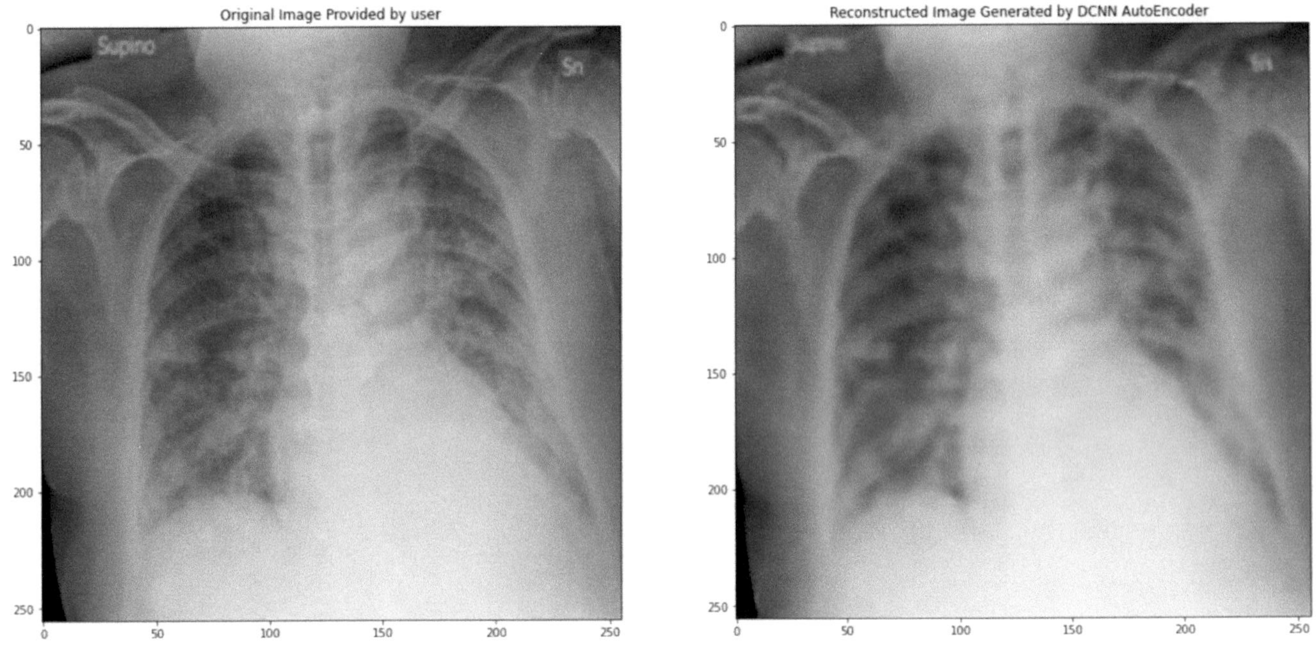

FIGURE 6.6 The stage training results that were obtained by the COVID-19 X-ray DCARN. (Obtained by training for 2,500 epochs; training being done on an Nvidia Tesla P100 GPU with Intel' s Xeon processors.)

In this chapter, we will delve into how we designed the image reconstruction system, which is based on the principle of preserving pixel intensities through a custom-designed deep convolutional auto-encoder infrastructure. This infrastructure takes an input X-ray image and produces the same image as output with minimal distortions, allowing us to gain insights into the various features concealed within the corresponding X-ray images. Figure 6.6 has been derived in Python during the designing of the architecture and testing the generation capabilities.

Based on the figure above, we can conclude that the DCARN, designed for X-ray image reconstruction of COVID-19 pneumonia, yielded satisfactory results. The images used for COVID-19 pneumonia reconstruction were obtained from the dataset presented in Chapters 3 and 4 of this book. However, the dataset for this chapter differs slightly.

In this chapter, we'll be working with images resized in a manner not commonly used by traditional machine learning engineers in Python. While working with CNNs, it's typical to resize images to dimensions like 32×32×3, 64×64×3, 128×128×3, and so on for improved accuracy. However, the main advantage of this AE application is the ability to work with dynamic image sizes. If readers wish to experiment with different dimensions, it won't be a complex task since we have proposed a solution that we will implement using pure Python with the assistance of TensorFlow and Numpy. The architecture has been designed in a functional manner to ensure usability with domain knowledge, and the name is simply an abbreviation representing the concept. In the following section, we will explore how to implement such a compound design combined with an AE for pneumonia image reconstruction.

6.4 THE DATA PREPROCESSING FOR THE DCARN

For all the applications, the data was used in an efficient way. We have proposed a nice system for converting the entire dataset into the Numpy arrays of the respective network. The libraries that were used are also very commonly used by data scientists, like Numpy for complex matrix manipulation, Matplotlib for plotting purpose, os for files handling in Python, glob for path flow control, and OpenCV for image preprocessing.

Python libraries:

```
"import numpy as np"
"import matplotlib.pyplot as plt"
"import tensorflow.keras as keras"
"import glob as glob"
"import cv2"
"from tqdm import tqdm as tqdm"
```

The data preprocessing stage begins here, the value of size can be changed to any number like 128, 256, 350, 720, 1080, and so on but yes for overall users the value of size must be kept between 200 and 500 for best possible results.

Python Code:

```
"from tensorflow.keras.preprocessing.image import img_to_
array"
"size = 256"

"image_list_1 = []"
"image_list_2 = []"
"image_list_3 = []"
"image_list_4 = []"

"image_path_1 = "
"for item in tqdm(sorted(glob.glob(image_path_1+"/*.*"))):"
    "image = cv2.imread(item, 1)"
    "img = cv2.cvtColor(image, cv2.COLOR_BGR2RGB)"
    "resized = cv2.resize(img, (size, size), cv2.INTER_LINEAR)"
    "image_list_1.append(img_to_array(resized))"

"image_path_2 = "
"for item in tqdm(sorted(glob.glob(image_path_2+"/*.*"))):"
    "image = cv2.imread(item, 1)"
    "img = cv2.cvtColor(image, cv2.COLOR_BGR2RGB)"
    "resized = cv2.resize(img, (size, size), cv2.INTER_LINEAR)"
    "image_list_2.append(img_to_array(resized))"

"image_path_3 = "
"for item in tqdm(sorted(glob.glob(image_path_3+"/*.*"))):"
    "image = cv2.imread(item, 1)"
    "img = cv2.cvtColor(image, cv2.COLOR_BGR2RGB)"
    "resized = cv2.resize(img, (size, size), cv2.INTER_LINEAR)"
    "image_list_3.append(img_to_array(resized))"

"image_path_4 = "
"for item in tqdm(sorted(glob.glob(image_path_4+"/*.*"))):"
    "image = cv2.imread(item, 1)"
    "img = cv2.cvtColor(image, cv2.COLOR_BGR2RGB)"
    "resized = cv2.resize(img, (size, size), cv2.INTER_LINEAR)"
    "image_list_4.append(img_to_array(resized))"

"list1 = np.reshape(image_list_1, (len(image_list_1), size,
size, 3))"
"list2 = np.reshape(image_list_2, (len(image_list_2), size,
size, 3))"
"list3 = np.reshape(image_list_3, (len(image_list_3), size,
size, 3))"
"list4 = np.reshape(image_list_4, (len(image_list_4), size,
size, 3))"

"np_array_1 = list1.astype('float32') / 255.0"
"np_array_2 = list2.astype('float32') / 255.0"
"np_array_3 = list3.astype('float32') / 255.0"
"np_array_4 = list4.astype('float32') / 255.0"

"print("Resizing Done")"
```

Upon completing the preprocessing steps mentioned above, the entire dataset that we will be working with will be converted into corresponding Numpy arrays for the training and validation procedures. The input shape for the proposed DCARN consists of four dimensions. The first dimension represents the batch size of images, or in simpler terms, how many images we want to use for training. The second, third, and fourth dimensions represent the shape of the images. In our case, the images were resized to a shape of [256, 256, 3] as depicted in Figure 6.7.

We can use four print statements to display the shapes of the training and validation Numpy arrays.

Python Code:

```
"print("The shape of the COVID-19-Pneumonia dataset is : {}".
format(np_array_1.shape))"
"print("The shape of the Non-COVID-19-Lung-Infection dataset
is : {}".format(np_array_2.shape))"
"print("The shape of the Normal-Lungs dataset is : {}".
format(np_array_3.shape))"
"print("The shape of the Viral
Pneumonia dataset is : {}".format(np_array_4.shape))"
```

Console Output:

```
The shape of the COVID-19-Pneumonia dataset is : (85, 256, 256, 3)
The shape of the Non-COVID-19-Lung-Infection dataset is : (83, 256, 256, 3)
The shape of the Normal-Lungs dataset is : (78, 256, 256, 3)
The shape of the Viral-Pneumonia dataset is : (82, 256, 256, 3)
```

FIGURE 6.7 The shapes formed for the data tensors on both training and validation data.

Thus, we have trained the entire architecture with around a total of 328 images (85 in the case of COVID-19 pneumonia, 83 in the case of non-COVID-19 lung infection, 78 belonging to the category of normal lungs, and 82 belonging to the category of viral pneumonia. The shapes of the Numpy arrays are as mentioned above, have four dimensions [X, Y, Z, W], where X represents the batch size, Y and Z represent the width and height of the images, and W represents the depth (1 means black and white images and 3 means color images).

6.5 THE DCARN IMPLEMENTATION USING TENSORFLOW IN PYTHON

Our implemented DCARN employs an encoder and decoder architecture that is somewhat equivalent to the VGG16 and VGG19 architectures. The encoder consists of multiple convolutional layers that aim to expand the channels of the input images using convolutional operations. Our inputs have a shape of [256, 256, 3], and after the first convolutional layers, the outputs become [256, 256, 64]. In other words, the number of channels changed from 3 to 64 due to the convolutional operations.

Following the convolution operations, we include max pooling 2D layers to help the network capture relevant hidden features present in the input image during training as depicted in Figure 6.8. We have designed the architecture in a functional manner to ensure the code's reusability. Generally, default hyperparameter values perform well, but sometimes tuning these hyperparameters can improve the network's performance slightly.

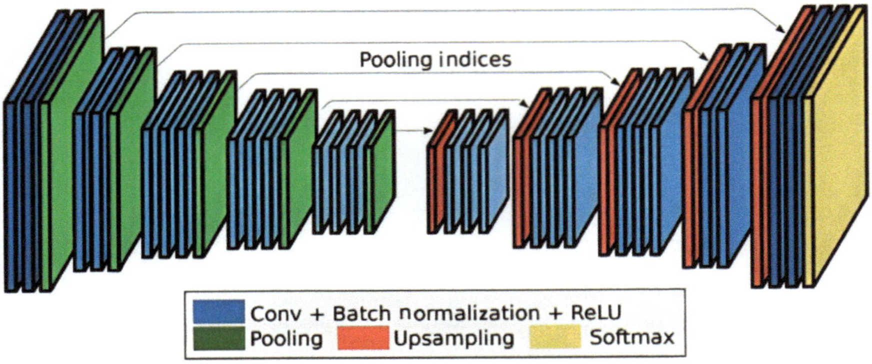

FIGURE 6.8 An auto-encoder architecture that follows the layered stack-like structure like the VGG16.

Python Code for the implementation of the DCARN:

```
"from keras.models import Model"
"from keras.layers import Input, Conv2D, MaxPooling2D,
UpSampling2D, concatenate, Conv2DTranspose,
BatchNormalization, Dropout, Lambda"
"from tensorflow.keras.optimizers import Adam, Adamax"
"from keras.layers import Activation, MaxPool2D, Concatenate"

#Convolutional block to be used in autoencoder and U-Net
"def conv_block(input, num_filters):"
    "x = Conv2D(num_filters, 3, padding="same")(input)"
    "x = BatchNormalization()(x)"   #Not in the original network.
    "x = Activation("relu")(x)"

    "x = Conv2D(num_filters, 3, padding="same")(x)"
    "x = BatchNormalization()(x)"  #Not in the original network
    "x = Activation("relu")(x)"

    "return x"

#Encoder block: Conv block followed by maxpooling
"def encoder_block(input, num_filters):"
    "x = conv_block(input, num_filters)"
    "p = MaxPool2D((2, 2))(x)"
    "return x, p"
#Decoder block for autoencoder (no skip connections)
"def decoder_block(input, num_filters):"
    "x = Conv2DTranspose(num_filters, (2, 2), strides=2,
padding="same")(input)"
```

```
    "x = conv_block(x, num_filters)"
    "return x"

#Encoder will be the same for Autoencoder and U-net
#We are getting both conv output and maxpool output for convenience.
#we will ignore conv output for Autoencoder. It acts as skip
connections for U-Net

"def build_encoder(input_image):"
    "s1, p1 = encoder_block(input_image, 64)"
    "s2, p2 = encoder_block(p1, 128)"
    "s3, p3 = encoder_block(p2, 256)"
    "s4, p4 = encoder_block(p3, 512)"

    #Bridge
    "encoded = conv_block(p4, 1024)"

    "return encoded"

#Decoder for Autoencoder ONLY.
"def build_decoder(encoded):"
    "d1 = decoder_block(encoded, 512)"
    "d2 = decoder_block(d1, 256)"
    "d3 = decoder_block(d2, 128)"
    "d4 = decoder_block(d3, 64)"

    "decoded = Conv2D(3, 3, padding="same", activation=
    "sigmoid")(d4)"
    "return decoded"

#Use encoder and decoder blocks to build the autoencoder.
"def build_autoencoder(input_shape):"
    "input_img = Input(shape=input_shape)"
    "autoencoder = Model(input_img, build_decoder(build_
encoder(input_img)))"
    "return(autoencoder)"

# Creating the corresponding DCARNs for the individual
feature extraction

"Model_1 = build_autoencoder((size, size, 3))" # The COVID-
19-Pneumonia X-ray DCARN
"Model_2 = build_autoencoder((size, size, 3))" # The Non-
COVID-19-Pneumonia X-ray DCARN
"Model_3 = build_autoencoder((size, size, 3))" # The Normal-
Lungs DCARN X-ray
"Model_4 = build_autoencoder((size, size, 3))" # The Viral-
Pneumonia X-ray DCARN

# print(Model_1.summary())
# print(Model_2.summary())
# print(Model_3.summary())
# print(Model_4.summary())

"X_train_1 = np_array_1[:70]"

"X_test_1 = np_array_1[70:]"
```

```
"print(X_train_1.shape, X_test_1.shape)"
"Model_1.compile(optimizer=keras.optimizers.Adamax(),
                loss='mean_squared_error',
                metrics=['accuracy','mae'])"

"Model_1_history = Model_1.fit(X_train_1,
                              X_train_1,
                              epochs=2500,
                              shuffle=True,
                              validation_data=(X_test_1, X_
                              test_1))"
```

The DCARN was trained with a Numpy array having the dimension of [70, 256, 256, 3] and was validated with a Numpy array having a shape of [15, 256, 256, 3]. The designed neural network architecture as depicted in Figure 6.9 is also provided below as console output as those who will be following till now can be able to get this particular result as output. Below provided output also helps the reader to understand the principle of dimensionality reduction using convolution operation along with max pooling.

```
Model: "model"
_________________________________________________________________
Layer (type)                  Output Shape              Param #
=================================================================
input_1 (InputLayer)          [(None, 256, 256, 3)]     0

conv2d (Conv2D)               (None, 256, 256, 64)      1792

batch_normalization (BatchN   (None, 256, 256, 64)      256
ormalization)

activation (Activation)       (None, 256, 256, 64)      0

conv2d_1 (Conv2D)             (None, 256, 256, 64)      36928

batch_normalization_1 (Batc   (None, 256, 256, 64)      256
hNormalization)

activation_1 (Activation)     (None, 256, 256, 64)      0

max_pooling2d (MaxPooling2D   (None, 128, 128, 64)      0
)

conv2d_2 (Conv2D)             (None, 128, 128, 128)     73856

batch_normalization_2 (Batc   (None, 128, 128, 128)     512
hNormalization)

activation_2 (Activation)     (None, 128, 128, 128)     0

conv2d_3 (Conv2D)             (None, 128, 128, 128)     147584

batch_normalization_3 (Batc   (None, 128, 128, 128)     512
hNormalization)
activation_3 (Activation)     (None, 128, 128, 128)     0

max_pooling2d_1 (MaxPooling   (None, 64, 64, 128)       0
2D)

conv2d_4 (Conv2D)             (None, 64, 64, 256)       295168

batch_normalization_4 (Batc   (None, 64, 64, 256)       1024
hNormalization)

activation_4 (Activation)     (None, 64, 64, 256)       0

conv2d_5 (Conv2D)             (None, 64, 64, 256)       590080

batch_normalization_5 (Batc   (None, 64, 64, 256)       1024
hNormalization)

activation_5 (Activation)     (None, 64, 64, 256)       0

max_pooling2d_2 (MaxPooling   (None, 32, 32, 256)       0
2D)

conv2d_6 (Conv2D)             (None, 32, 32, 512)       1180160

batch_normalization_6 (Batc   (None, 32, 32, 512)       2048
hNormalization)

activation_6 (Activation)     (None, 32, 32, 512)       0

conv2d_7 (Conv2D)             (None, 32, 32, 512)       2359808

batch_normalization_7 (Batc   (None, 32, 32, 512)       2048
hNormalization)

activation_7 (Activation)     (None, 32, 32, 512)       0

max_pooling2d_3 (MaxPooling   (None, 16, 16, 512)       0
2D)

conv2d_8 (Conv2D)             (None, 16, 16, 1024)      4719616

batch_normalization_8 (Batc   (None, 16, 16, 1024)      4096
hNormalization)

activation_8 (Activation)     (None, 16, 16, 1024)      0

conv2d_9 (Conv2D)             (None, 16, 16, 1024)      9438208

batch_normalization_9 (Batc   (None, 16, 16, 1024)      4096
hNormalization)

activation_9 (Activation)     (None, 16, 16, 1024)      0

conv2d_transpose (Conv2DTra   (None, 32, 32, 512)       2097664
nspose)

conv2d_10 (Conv2D)            (None, 32, 32, 512)       2359808

batch_normalization_10 (Bat   (None, 32, 32, 512)       2048
chNormalization)

activation_10 (Activation)    (None, 32, 32, 512)       0

conv2d_11 (Conv2D)            (None, 32, 32, 512)       2359808

batch_normalization_11 (Bat   (None, 32, 32, 512)       2048
chNormalization)

activation_11 (Activation)    (None, 32, 32, 512)       0

conv2d_transpose_1 (Conv2DT   (None, 64, 64, 256)       524544
ranspose)

conv2d_12 (Conv2D)            (None, 64, 64, 256)       590080
batch_normalization_12 (Bat   (None, 64, 64, 256)       1024
chNormalization)

activation_12 (Activation)    (None, 64, 64, 256)       0

conv2d_13 (Conv2D)            (None, 64, 64, 256)       590080

batch_normalization_13 (Bat   (None, 64, 64, 256)       1024
chNormalization)

activation_13 (Activation)    (None, 64, 64, 256)       0

conv2d_transpose_2 (Conv2DT   (None, 128, 128, 128)     131200
ranspose)

conv2d_14 (Conv2D)            (None, 128, 128, 128)     147584

batch_normalization_14 (Bat   (None, 128, 128, 128)     512
chNormalization)

activation_14 (Activation)    (None, 128, 128, 128)     0

conv2d_15 (Conv2D)            (None, 128, 128, 128)     147584

batch_normalization_15 (Bat   (None, 128, 128, 128)     512
chNormalization)

activation_15 (Activation)    (None, 128, 128, 128)     0

conv2d_transpose_3 (Conv2DT   (None, 256, 256, 64)      32832
ranspose)

conv2d_16 (Conv2D)            (None, 256, 256, 64)      36928

batch_normalization_16 (Bat   (None, 256, 256, 64)      256
chNormalization)

activation_16 (Activation)    (None, 256, 256, 64)      0
```

FIGURE 6.9 The detailed architecture of the proposed network and the corresponding training steps.

As we can observe, the entire network is sufficiently deep to capture crucial hidden feature representations related to the provided input images, specifically X-ray images of pneumonia. Our designed network consists of numerous convolutional layers paired with max pooling to enhance optimization during training. Unlike in our previous chapters, we employed a slightly different optimizer known as Adamax optimization. Through experimentation, we found that using optimizers like Adam, Adamax, and Nadam tends to yield the best results. The DCARN architecture comprises a total of 63 layers for X-ray image reconstruction.

6.6 THE RESULT ANALYSIS BY PLOTTING PERFORMANCE METRICS GRAPHS

We have created the same code that we use for tracing the training metrics. The code will help us to plot the corresponding training and validation mean squared errors, as we are performing the task of image reconstruction, so we proposed to use the mean squared error as the loss function for the problem. We have also tried to plot the accuracy metrics but as we have trained for a longer period of time, so the graphs are a bit squeezed. We have used Matplotlib significantly for plotting the graphs as we have seen in Chapter 3 and Chapter 4. Figure 6.10 depicts the model training and validation performance graphs.

Python Code:

```
"import matplotlib.pyplot as plt"

"f, (ax1, ax2) = plt.subplots(1, 2, figsize=(15, 5))"
"t = f.suptitle('CNN Performance', fontsize=12)"
"f.subplots_adjust(top=0.85, wspace=0.3)"

"max_epoch = len(Model_1_history.history['accuracy'])+1"
"epoch_list = list(range(1,max_epoch))"
"ax1.plot(epoch_list, Model_1_history.history['accuracy'],
label='Train Accuracy')"
"ax1.plot(epoch_list, Model_1_history.history['mae'], label=
'Training Mean Absolute Error')"
"ax1.set_xticks(np.arange(1, max_epoch, 5))"
"ax1.set_ylabel('Accuracy and MAE Values')"
"ax1.set_xlabel('Epoch')"
"ax1.set_title('Accuracy VS Mean Absolute Error')"
"l1 = ax1.legend(loc="best")"

"ax2.plot(epoch_list, Model_1_history.history['loss'],
label='Train Loss')"
"ax2.plot(epoch_list, Model_1_history.history['mae'], label=
'Training Mean Absolute Error')"
"ax2.set_xticks(np.arange(1, max_epoch, 5))"
"ax2.set_ylabel('Loss and MAE Values')"
"ax2.set_xlabel('Epoch')"
"ax2.set_title('Loss VS Mean Absolute Error')"
"l2 = ax2.legend(loc="best")"
```

Console Output:

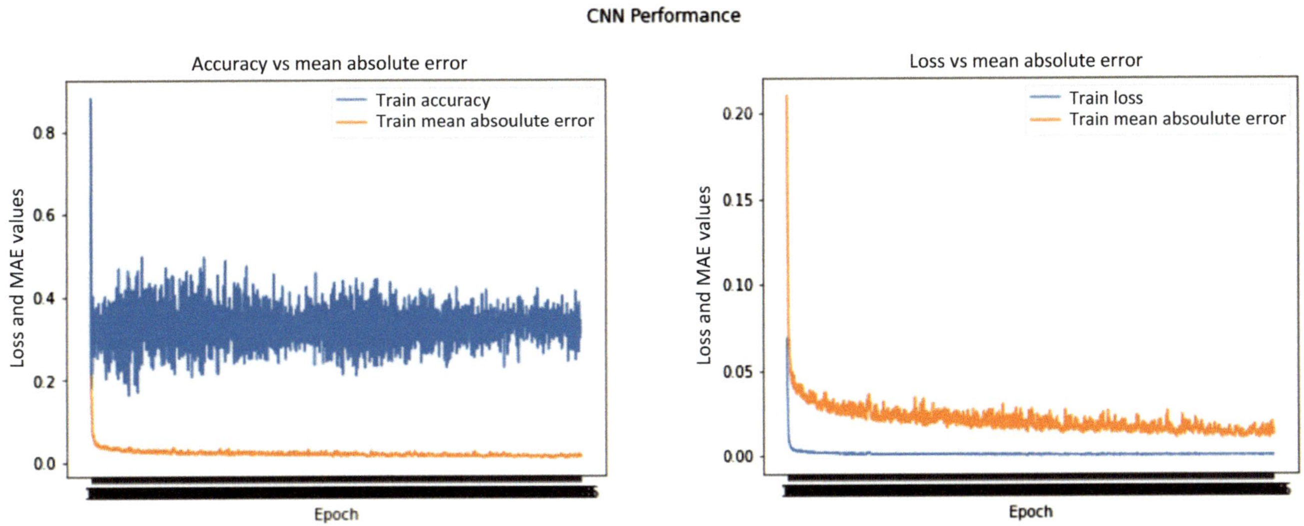

FIGURE 6.10 The performance graphs of the proposed DCARN.

As we have seen the graphs of the proposed auto-encoder system tend to gradually decrease, we can conclude that the training of the network was done properly. In deep learning, the system we create tends to depend on the hyperparameters a lot. By changing the hyperparameters, a bit, one can easily optimize any neural networks. In the case of the DCARN, the hyperparameter that we have tuned is the main proposal of the system's optimization and thus this optimization can be overcome using the traditional principles of machine learning and Bayes' theorem. The main hyperparameters of the proposed system, the DCARN, are the values of the units of each convolutional layers of the AE. In our case we have used the default values for the demonstration. In the coming section we will discuss how we can use the trained model for performing predictions on real time. We have created a function for the prediction of the features that are captured during the reconstruction of the input. The entire system was capable of reconstructing many inputs to their corresponding outputs and thus while performing the reconstruction, the network learns the hidden features that are present in the input as depicted in Figure 6.11. The function that we have created uses some important Python libraries, like Numpy, Tensorflow, and Matplotlib.

Python code for inference on the trained model upon the test dataset:

```
"pred = model_1.predict(img_array_1)"
"fig, ax = plt.subplots(figsize=(20,20))"
"plt.subplot(1,2,1)"
"plt.imshow(img)"
"plt.title('Original Image Provided by user')"
"plt.subplot(1,2,2)"
"plt.imshow(pred[0].reshape(SIZE,SIZE,3))"
"plt.title('Reconstructed Image Generated by DCNN
AutoEncoder')"
"plt.show()"
```

Console Output:

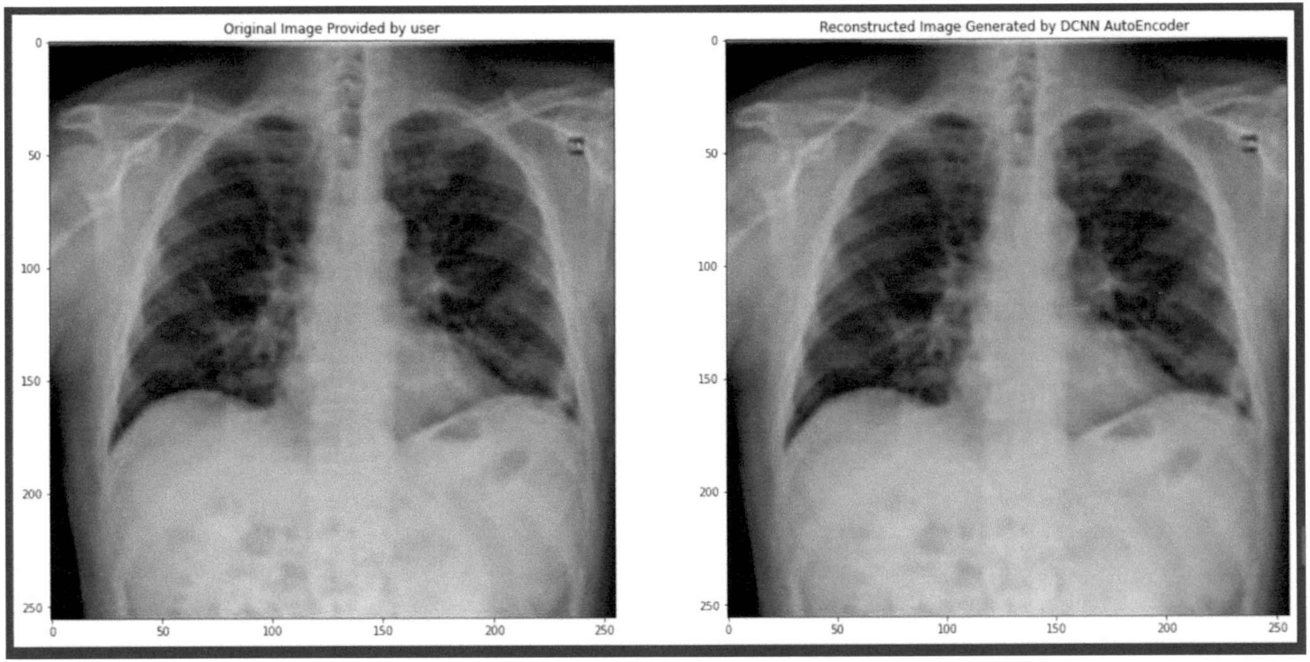

FIGURE 6.11 Console output for reconstructed image.

Hence, the system effectively executed the reconstruction of the input image, and we can attribute this success to the design of the AE. The original image provided was resized to dimensions of 256×256×3, and the reconstructed output also remained at the same size of 256×256×3. Consequently, the network acquired an understanding of various features present in the provided image of COVID-19 pneumonia X-ray.

In the subsequent section, we've included a segment of Python code that enables us to visualize the outputs of various convolutional and max pooling layers. This aids in enhancing our comprehension of how CNNs operate. Although CNNs are often seen as black boxes, AEs offer a means to gain insight into their inner workings. During the process of image reconstruction using an auto-encoder, we've developed a function that facilitates the visualization of features learned by the layers within the auto-encoder depicted in Figure 6.12. This function enables us to plot the feature outputs of these layers. Key Python libraries such as Matplotlib, Numpy, and Tensorflow have played pivotal roles in drawing these final conclusions.

Python code for plotting the different features:

```
#Model before training... random weights.. for comparison
"model2 = build_autoencoder(img.shape)"
"my_model = model_1"
"import warnings"
"warnings.filterwarnings('ignore')"
#set intermediate representations for all layers in
the model
# except for the first - as it is an input layer
"outputs = [layer.output for layer in my_model.layers[1:]]"

"model_for_visualization = Model(inputs = my_model.input,
outputs = outputs)"

#Generate random image to be used as input
# img = np.uint8(np.random.uniform(120, 200, (256, 256,
3)))/255

# input_img = np.expand_dims(img, axis=0)
"input_img = img_array_1"
"feature_maps = model_for_visualization.predict(input_img)"

"layer_num = 17" # Depth of layer...
"for i in range(layer_num):"
    "print("The output features of the {} layer is {} ".
    format(i, "\n"))"
    "square = 10"
    "ix = 1"
    "fig, ax1 = plt.subplots(figsize=(15,15))"
    "for _ in range(square):"
        "for _ in range(square):"
            # specify subplot and turn of axis
            "ax = plt.subplot(square, square, ix)"
            "ax.set_xticks([])"
            "ax.set_yticks([])"
```

```
            # plot filter channel in grayscale
            "plt.imshow(feature_maps[layer_num][0, :, :, ix-1])"
            "ix += 1"
    # show the figure
    "plt.show()"
```

Console Output:

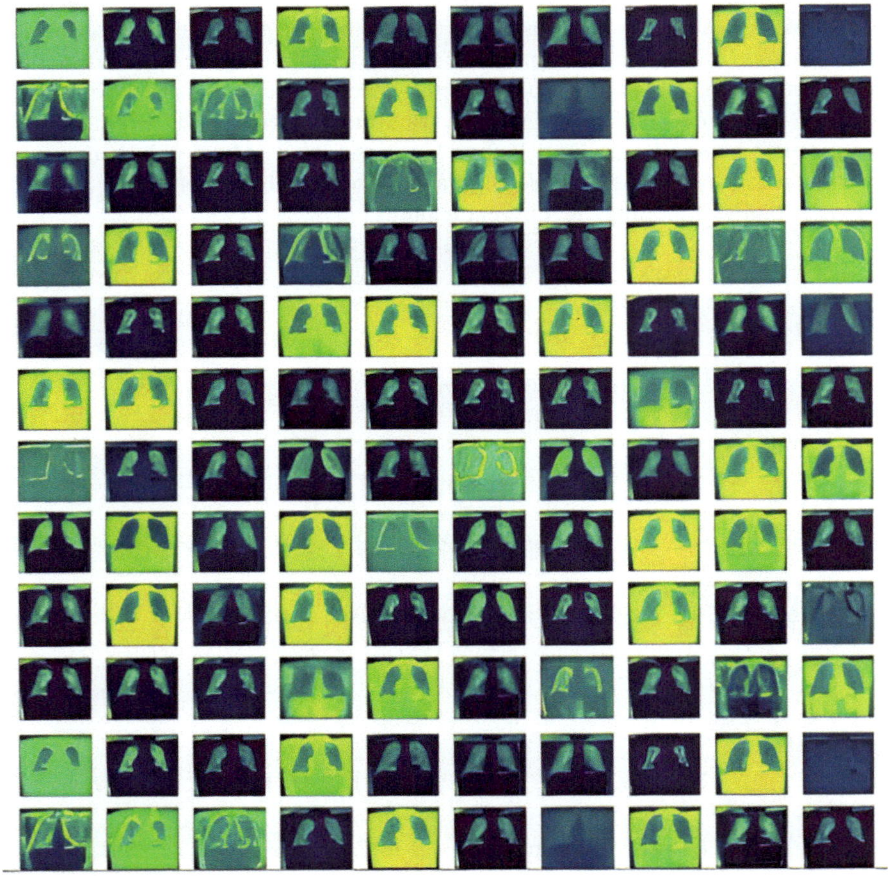

FIGURE 6.12 Consol output of feature map.

6.7 CONCLUSION

Consequently, upon executing the final plotting function, we obtain visual representations of the feature outputs from various convolutional layers within the AE. These feature maps serve as critical components in determining images of distinct categories. This process provides a clearer understanding of how CNNs operate when processing images. The features that convolutional neural networks extract during image processing are akin to the reconstruction process employed by a convolutional auto-encoder network. The proposed system, DCARN, serves as a tool to comprehend the inner workings of convolutional neural networks through image reconstruction. This experiment sheds light on the fact that CNNs excel in various image recognition tasks due to their ability to extract features from images. Consequently, computer vision applications greatly benefit from the capabilities of convolutional neural networks.

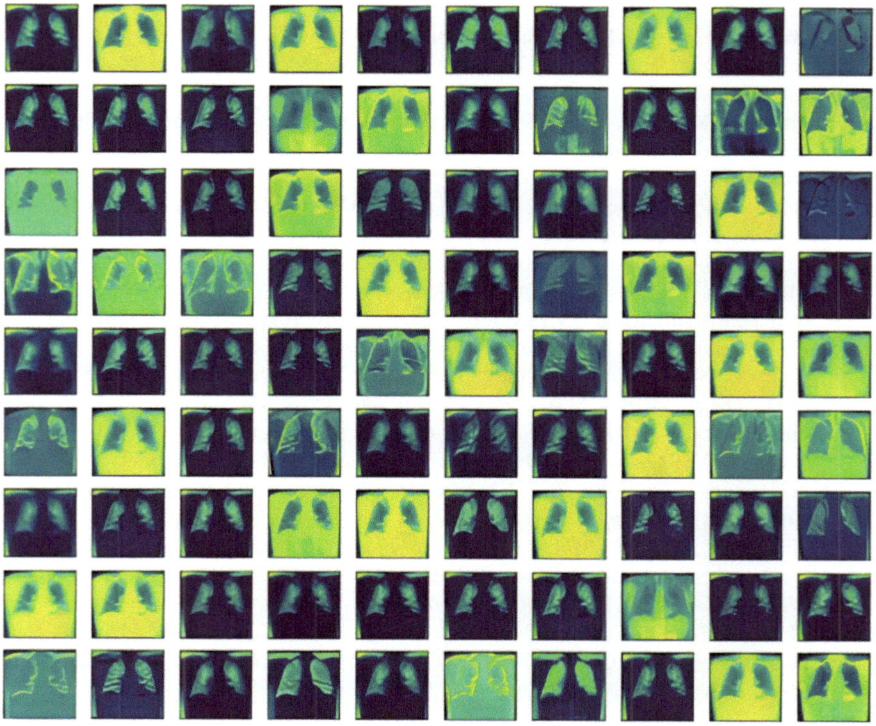

FIGURE 6.13 The feature maps that were generated by deeper layers of the auto-encoder.

Figure 6.13 illustrates that as we delve deeper into the neural network, the features extracted become increasingly complex. DCARN, with its 60+ layers, provides an opportunity to plot and compare these features with various input images, facilitating a better understanding of the inner functions of CNNs. It is evident that deeper CNNs excel at capturing intricate features, which, although challenging for the human eye to discern, greatly enhance the network's ability to perform domain-specific image recognition tasks.

REFERENCES

1. Li, Z., Liu, F., Yang, W., Peng, S. and Zhou, J., 2021. A survey of convolutional neural networks: analysis, applications, and prospects. *IEEE Transactions on Neural Networks and Learning Systems.*
2. Kalchbrenner, N., Grefenstette, E. and Blunsom, P., 2014. A convolutional neural network for modelling sentences. *arXiv preprint arXiv:1404.2188.*
3. O'Shea, K. and Nash, R., 2015. An introduction to convolutional neural networks. *arXiv preprint arXiv:1511.08458.*
4. Wiatowski, T. and Bölcskei, H., 2017. A mathematical theory of deep convolutional neural networks for feature extraction. *IEEE Transactions on Information Theory*, 64(3), pp. 1845–1866.
5. Weimer, D., Scholz-Reiter, B. and Shpitalni, M., 2016. Design of deep convolutional neural network architectures for automated feature extraction in industrial inspection. *CIRP Annals*, 65(1), pp. 417–420.
6. Yang, A., Yang, X., Wu, W., Liu, H. and Zhuansun, Y., 2019. Research on feature extraction of tumor image based on convolutional neural network. *IEEE Access*, 7, pp. 24204–24213.
7. Aslan, M.F., Unlersen, M.F., Sabanci, K. and Durdu, A., 2021. CNN-based transfer learning–BiLSTM network: A novel approach for COVID-19 infection detection. *Applied Soft Computing*, 98, p. 106912.
8. Monshi, M.M.A., Poon, J., Chung, V. and Monshi, F.M., 2021. CovidXrayNet: Optimizing data augmentation and CNN hyperparameters for improved COVID-19 detection from CXR. *Computers in Biology and Medicine*, 133, p. 104375.
9. Rehman, N.U., Zia, M.S., Meraj, T., Rauf, H.T., Damaševičius, R., El-Sherbeeny, A.M. and El-Meligy, M.A., 2021. A self-activated CNN approach for multi-class chest-related COVID-19 detection. *Applied Sciences*, 11(19), p. 9023.
10. Aslan, M.F., Sabanci, K., Durdu, A. and Unlersen, M.F., 2022. COVID-19 diagnosis using state-of-the-art CNN architecture features and Bayesian optimization. *Computers in Biology and Medicine.*
11. Islam, M.Z., Islam, M.M. and Asraf, A., 2020. A combined deep CNN-LSTM network for the detection of novel coronavirus (COVID-19) using X-ray images. *Informatics in Medicine Unlocked*, 20, p. 100412.
12. Shah, V., Keniya, R., Shridharani, A., Punjabi, M., Shah, J. and Mehendale, N., 2021. Diagnosis of COVID-19 using CT scan images and deep learning techniques. *Emergency Radiology*, 28(3), pp. 497–505.

7 Super Resolution Generative Adversarial Neural Network (SR-GANN) with Bi-Modal Multi-Perceptron Layers for Medical X-Ray Images

7.1 INTRODUCTION

In this chapter, we are going to explore how deep learning can be used to generate new images, specifically by delving into the realm of Generative Adversarial Networks (GANs) [1]. When it comes to data classification in deep learning, conventional techniques like artificial neural networks (ANNs), convolutional neural networks (CNNs), and recurrent neural networks (RNNs) are often employed. However, for tasks involving image generation, these traditional neural networks may fall short. That's where GANs come into play.

GANs consist of two neural networks that engage in a competitive learning process to produce more realistic and better-quality results. The first network, known as the generator, is responsible for creating new data samples. The second network, called the discriminator, is tasked with distinguishing between generated data samples and real ones. The generator continually strives to generate detailed samples that are so convincing that the discriminator cannot tell them the difference from real data. On the other hand, the discriminator aims to correctly identify whether a given sample is generated or real data. Both networks are trained simultaneously, and the generator attempts to deceive the discriminator by generating increasingly realistic data.

The ultimate goal of the generator is to produce data samples that are virtually indistinguishable from real ones. GANs operate in an adversarial manner, with the generator and discriminator working against each other to improve their respective performances.

The architecture of a GAN typically consists of two main components: the generator network and the discriminator network. The generator, when trained on a specific dataset, becomes capable of generating entirely new images from that domain. To ensure the generated images meet the required standards, the discriminator is responsible for classifying whether an image is generated by the generator or it is a real one.

DOI: 10.1201/9781003456476-7

The key to successful image generation with GANs lies in the adversarial training of the system over extended periods of time. GANs can yield exceptional results when provided with sufficient training time. In summary, GANs are a powerful deep learning technique used for generating images by training a generator network to create realistic samples that can fool a discriminator network. This adversarial training process is key to achieving high-quality image generation.

7.2 GENERATIVE ADVERSARIAL NEURAL NETWORKS

GANs are indeed a fascinating development in the field of deep learning. They consist of two distinct neural networks that collaborate in a unique way to achieve a specific goal.

- Generator: The generator network, as the name suggests, is responsible for creating new data, often in the form of images. It learns to generate data that resembles existing data. Initially, its generated data might not be very convincing, but it improves over time through training.
- Discriminator: The discriminator network, on the other hand, serves as a critic. Its job is to distinguish between real data (e.g., real images) and the data produced by the generator. It starts by being rather poor at this task but becomes more proficient through training.

The core idea of GANs is that these two networks are trained simultaneously and are in a constant competition. As the generator gets better at producing data that resembles real data, the discriminator must also improve to distinguish between real data and generated data. This adversarial process continues until the generator becomes so skilled at creating realistic data that the discriminator can hardly tell the difference.

This unique architecture allows GANs to generate data, including images, music, and even text, that can be remarkably realistic and often indistinguishable from human-generated content. GANs have found applications in a wide range of fields, including image generation, style transfer, data augmentation, and even drug discovery (Figures 7.1 and 7.2).

While both networks were trained using identical datasets, they were never exposed to duplicate images. The primary objective of the generator is to closely align the generated images with real ones, striving for maximum similarity. Conversely, the discriminator's primary role is to identify disparities between authentic and counterfeit images.

Figure 7.3 presents the entire block diagram of the GANN. The generator network is denoted by G and the discriminator is denoted by D. The input for the generator is the latent space dimension and the input for the discriminator is the generator's generated samples along with real samples. Thus, GANN can be treated as the combination of two neural networks. The architecture of the generator and the discriminator changes from application to application.

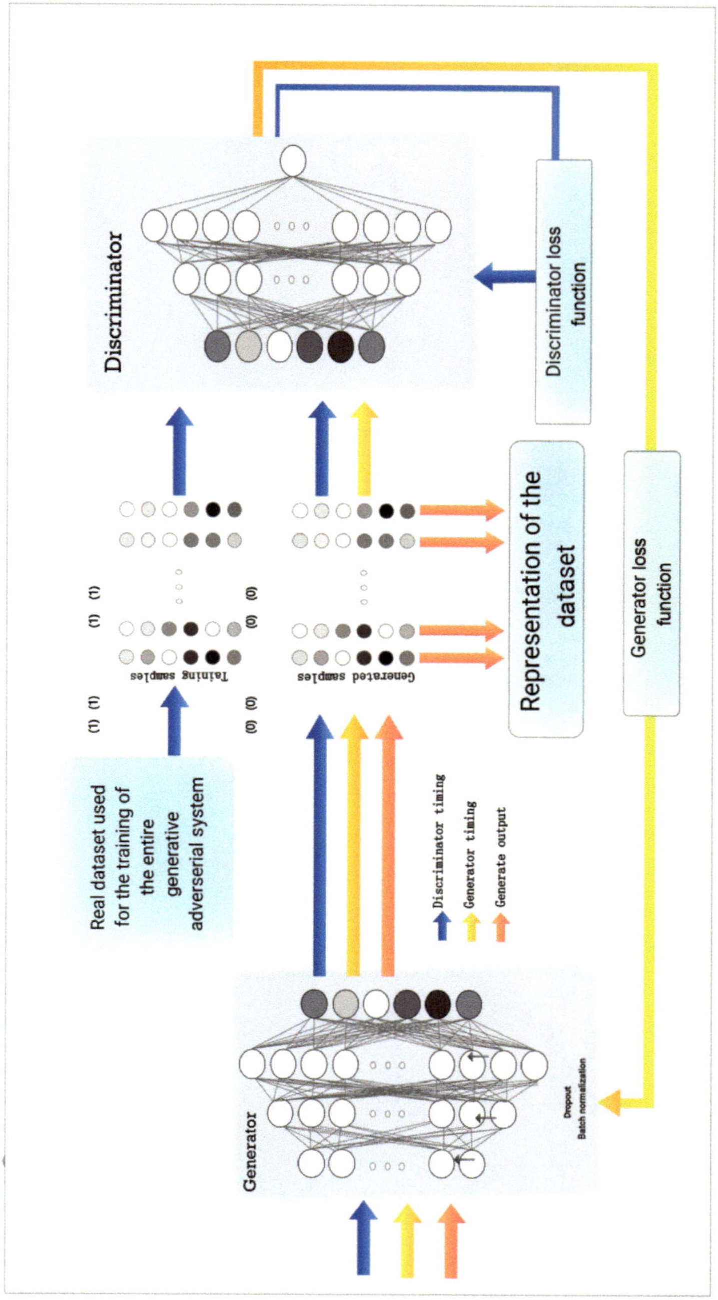

FIGURE 7.1 Block diagram of a generative adversarial neural network with artificial neural network generator and discriminator.

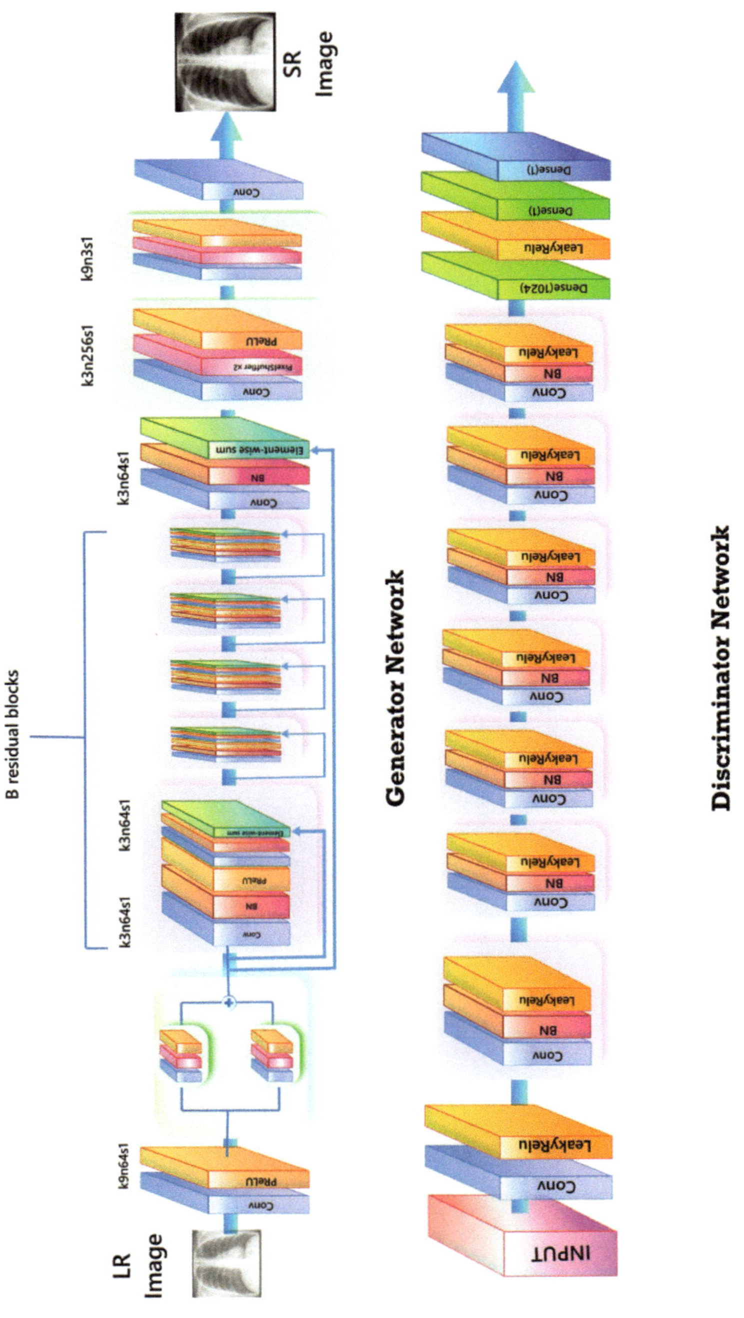

FIGURE 7.2 Our proposed super resolution generative adversarial neural network with residual generator layers and adaptive optimizations as well.

This competition between the two networks helps them learn to create more realistic images. GANs are designed to mimic high-level human cognitive functions (like the ability to recognize faces or scenes), and have been used to create new images of faces, cars, and animals that are realistic enough to fool humans. The researchers in this study wanted to see if they could improve the realism of existing GANs by training a GAN using images of eyes. Previous research on GANs has shown that they have difficulty generating realistic images of eyes, so if the researchers can train a GAN using eye images, it could be a step toward creating more realistic images of faces, which could help in developing new anti-spoofing authentication systems. The researchers built a dataset of 10,000 pictures of human eyes from various angles and lighting conditions. They then used the dataset to train three different GANs: one using only eye images as input data, one using only facial data as input data, and one using equal amounts of both eye and facial data. The researchers found that GANs trained on both eye and face image datasets had improved ability when generating new eye images than when trained on only face image datasets. Additionally, the researchers found that their GANs were able to learn how to generate a greater variety of eye shapes than those previously reported in research on GANs. The authors suggest that this demonstrates that incorporating non-face datasets into GANs can help them generate a wider variety of realistic images. Their findings may also suggest that incorporating more non-face image datasets into future studies on GANs could lead to better results for creating realistic face images as well.

7.2.1 Mathematical Modeling of Generative Adversarial Neural Network

In the realm of mathematical modeling for deep learning algorithms, the entire process is often referred to as a "Black Box" due to its empirical nature. The mathematical formulation of any GAN relies on the design of loss functions employed during the training process. GANs belong to the category of generative models, designed to uncover the underlying distribution of a data generation process through a dynamic interplay between a generator and a discriminator.

As previously introduced, GANs involve two models, namely, the generator and the discriminator, which undergo training. The discriminator's primary role is to distinguish between generated and authentic data samples, while the generator's objective is to confound the discriminator by producing data that is both realistic and convincing. GANs can be conceptualized as a cooperative effort between these two models, each equipped with its own unique loss function. In the following section, we will aim to provide an intuitive understanding of the loss function associated with each of these models.

7.2.2 Notation for GANN

To avoid any potential confusion, let us establish some notation that will be consistently utilized.

x: **Real data**
z: **Latent vector**

G(z): **Fake data**
D(x): **Discriminator's evaluation of real data**
D(G(z)): **Discriminator's evaluation of fake data**
Error (a, b): **Error between** a **and b**

As a result, the notations above are used to determine the final mathematical model of the GAN. The main concept is the formation of loss functions for proper training of the entire GANN, and the generator attempts to generate appropriate images through adversarial training. The generator outperforms the discriminator by attempting to improve its ability to generate new images through adversarial training.

7.2.3 The Discriminator

The discriminator's goal is to correctly label generated images as false while labeling empirical data points as true. As a result, we could consider the following to be the discriminator's loss function:

$$LD=Error(D(x),1)+Error(D(G(z)),0) \tag{7.1}$$

In this case, we're using a very broad, unspecific notation for error to refer to a function that informs us the distance or difference between two operating parameters. (If this immediately reminded you of something like cross entropy or Kullback–Leibler divergence, you're on the right track.)

7.2.4 The Generator

We can proceed with the generator in the same manner as for the discriminator. The generator's goal is to confuse the discriminator as much as possible so that it labels generated images as true.

$$LG=Error(D(G(z)),1) \tag{7.2}$$

The important thing to remember here is that a loss function is something we want to minimize. In the case of the generator, it should strive to minimize the difference between 1 and the discriminator's evaluation of the generated fake data.

7.2.5 Binary Cross Entropy

Binary cross entropy is a common loss function used in binary classification problems. Let's go over the cross-entropy formula again for a quick refresher:

$$H(p, q)=Ex{\sim}p(x)[-\log q(x)] \tag{7.3}$$

In classification tasks, the random variable is discrete. Hence, the expectation can be expressed as a summation.

$$H(p, q)=-\Sigma x{\in}\chi p(x)\log q(x) \tag{7.4}$$

We can simplify this expression even further in the case of binary cross entropy since there are only two labels: zero and one.

$$H\ (y, y^\wedge) = -\Sigma y \log(y^\wedge) + (1-y) \log(1-y^\wedge) \tag{7.5}$$

This is the error function that we referred to in the preceding sections. Binary cross entropy accomplishes our goal by measuring how different two distributions are in the context of binary classification of determining whether an input data point is true or false. When applied to the loss functions in (7.1),

$$LD = -\Sigma x \in \chi,\ z \in \zeta \log(D(x)) + \log(1-D(G(z))) \tag{7.6}$$

We can do the same for (7.2):

$$LG = -\Sigma z \in \zeta \log(D(G(z)) \tag{7.7}$$

We now have two loss functions to train the generator and discriminator. It is worth noting that the loss function of the generator is small if D(G(z)) is close to 1, because log (1) = 0. This is exactly the type of behavior we want from the generator's loss function. With a similar approach, it is easy to see the cogency of (7.6).

7.2.6 Minor Caveats

The original paper by Goodfellow presents a slightly different version of the two loss functions derived above.

$$\mathrm{Max}(D)\{\log(D(x)) + \log(1-D(G(z)))\} \tag{7.8}$$

The distinction between equations (7.6) and (7.8) primarily lies in the sign and the objective of minimizing or maximizing a specific quantity. Equation (7.6) formulates the function as a loss function to be minimized, while the original formulation in equation (7.8) presents it as a maximization problem, with a sign reversal. Goodfellow characterizes equation (7.8) as a min-max game, where the discriminator aims to maximize the given quantity while the generator pursues the opposite objective. In other words,

$$\mathrm{Min}(G)\max(D)\{\log(D(x)) + \log(1-D(G(z)))\} \tag{7.9}$$

The min-max formulation provides a concise representation of the adversarial relationship between the generator and the discriminator. However, in practical implementations, we establish distinct loss functions for both the generator and the discriminator, as illustrated earlier. This distinction arises from the fact that the gradient of the function $y = \log x$ is more pronounced near $x = 0$ than for the function $y = \log(1 - x)$. Consequently, optimizing log(D(G(z))) or, equivalently, minimizing log(D(G(z))), results in swifter and more substantial enhancements to the generator's performance compared to the task of minimizing log (1 – D(G(z))).

7.2.7 Model Optimization

Having established the loss functions for both the generator and the discriminator, we can now employ mathematical techniques to address the optimization problem, which involves determining the optimal parameters for these components to minimize their respective loss functions. In practice, this translates to the training process of the model. When training a GAN, it is customary to train one component at a time. Specifically, during the training of the discriminator, we assume that the generator's parameters remain fixed. The amount of interest can be represented as a function of GG and DD. This is referred to as the value function:

$$V(G, D) = E_{x \sim pdata}[\log(D(x))] + E_{z \sim pz}[\log(1 - D(G(z)))] \tag{7.10}$$

In reality, we're more involved in the generator's distribution than pz. As little more than a result, let's define a new variable, $y = G(z)$, and rewrite the value function with this substitution:

$$V(G, D) = E_{x \sim pdata}[\log(D(x))] + E_{y \sim pg}[\log(1 - D(y))]$$

$$= \int_{x \in \chi} pdata(x)\log(D(x)) + pg(x)\log(1 - D(x))\, dx \tag{7.11}$$

The objective of the discriminator is to maximize the value function V (G, D). We can observe, by taking a partial derivative of V (G, D) with respect to $D(x)$, that the optimal discriminator, denoted as $D(x)$, is achieved when

$$\frac{p_{data}(x)}{D(x)} - \frac{p_g(x)}{1 - D(x)} = 0 \tag{7.12}$$

Rearranging (7.12), we get

$$D^*(x) = \frac{p_{data}(x)}{p_{data}(x) + p_g(x)} \tag{7.13}$$

This represents the optimal discriminator condition. It's important to note that this formula aligns with our intuition: if a sample x is highly authentic, we would anticipate $pdata(x)$ to approach 1 and $pg(x)$ to approach 0. In this scenario, the ideal discriminator would assign it a score of 1. Conversely, for a generated sample $x = G(z)$, we would expect the optimal discriminator to assign a score of 0, as pdata(G(z)) should be close to zero. To train the generator, we assume that the discriminator is held constant and we proceed with the analysis of the value function. To start, we substitute the previously mentioned result, equation (7.12), into the value function and observe the outcomes.

$$\begin{aligned} V(G,D^*) &= E_{x\sim p_{data}}\left[\log\left(D^*(x)\right)\right] + E_{x\sim p_g}\left[\log\left(1-D^*(x)\right)\right] \\ &= E_{x\sim p_{data}}\left[\log\frac{p_{data}(x)}{p_{data}(x)+p_g(x)}\right] + E_{x\sim p_g}\left[\log\frac{p_g(x)}{p_{data}(x)+p_g(x)}\right] \end{aligned}$$

To proceed from here, we need a little bit of inspiration.

$$\begin{aligned} V(G,D^*) &= E_{x\sim p_{data}}\left[\log\frac{p_{data}(x)}{p_{data}(x)+p_g(x)}\right] + E_{x\sim p_g}\left[\log\frac{p_g(x)}{p_{data}(x)+p_g(x)}\right] \\ &= -\log 4 + E_{x\sim p_{data}}\left[\log p_{data}(x) - \log\frac{p_{data}(x)+p_g(x))}{2}\right] \\ &\quad + E_{x\sim p_g}\left[\log p_g(x) - \log\frac{p_{data}(x)+p_g(x))}{2}\right] \end{aligned} \tag{7.14}$$

Don't be concerned if this appears confusing; you're not alone. Essentially, we are utilizing logarithmic properties to introduce a -log4 that wasn't present before. Once we obtain this value, we need to make adjustments to the terms in the expectation, particularly by dividing the denominator by 2.

7.2.8 Why Was This Necessary?

The magic here is that we can now interpret the expectations as Kullback–Leibler divergence:

$$V(G,D^*) = -\log 4 + D_{KL}\left(p_{data} \,||\, \frac{p_{data}+p_g}{2}\right) + D_{KL}\left(p_g \,||\, \frac{p_g+p_g}{2}\right) \tag{7.15}$$

And it is here that we re-encounter the Jensen Shannon divergence, which is defined as

$$J(P,Q) = \frac{1}{2}\left(D(P \,||\, R) + D(Q \,||\, R)\right)$$

where $R = \frac{1}{2}(P+Q)$. This means that the expression in (7.15) can be expressed as a JS divergence:

$$V(G,D^*) = -\log 4 + 2 \cdot D_{JS}\left(p_{data} \parallel p_g\right)$$

The conclusion of this analysis is straightforward: when training the generator to minimize the value function V, we aim to minimize the JS divergence between the data distribution and the distribution of generated examples (G, D). This aligns with our expectations: we want the generator to effectively learn the underlying data distribution from the training examples. In essence, pg and pdata should closely resemble each other. To create a convincing model distribution pg, the generator GG must excel at emulating pdata. Since the publication of Goodfellow's work, various researchers have introduced and studied additional GAN models.

7.3 THE IMAGE SUPER RESOLUTION GENERATIVE ADVERSARIAL NEURAL NETWORK FOR SUPER RESOLUTION OF X-RAY IMAGES OF AROUND 5,000 PATIENTS

SR-GANN is a deep learning algorithm that improves image resolution by employing GAN. The algorithm is trained on a set of low-resolution images and their high-resolution counterparts [2, 3]. The low-resolution images are fed into a generator network, where they are upscaled to the high-resolution version. A discriminator network is then used to try to differentiate between the upscaled images and the true high-resolution images. The generator network is trained to deceive the discriminator, learning to generate high-resolution images from low-resolution images. SR-GAN GANs have previously been used to generate fake image data and text like proposed in [4–6]. They did, however, work best with data that was already present in the dataset. The high-resolution versions of the images were not available in this case. Nvidia researchers developed SR-GANN to allow GANs to be trained on real images rather than on simulated ones. The GAN is set up to generate images of the size that the neural network anticipates seeing. This is accomplished by scaling the low-resolution images to roughly twice their original size. After that, the low-resolution images are upscaled using a standard algorithm, such as bicubic or bilinear interpolation. The upscaled images are fed into the generator network, which produces high-resolution images. The discriminator network learns to differentiate between high-resolution images and true high-resolution images. The generator learns to generate upscaled images that are pragmatic enough to fool the discriminator in the process. The GAN is trained by alternately training the discriminator and the generator to distinguish between low-resolution and high-resolution images [7, 8]. This method works well for images [9, 10], with a lot of texture, like photographs. However, for images with little texture, such as line drawings, the results are not convincing enough to fool you into thinking the low-resolution images are of high resolution.

7.3.1 The Generator Can be Trained in Two Ways

7.3.1.1 Contrastive Divergence

The discriminator and the generator are trained concurrently while the binary cross entropy loss function is maximized. This is accomplished by backpropagating through the gradients of both networks to determine their contribution to each network's error and calculating the difference between these values. This distinction is known as a contrastive divergence, and it is used to update both networks.

7.3.1.2 Adversarial Training

The discriminator has been trained to maximize the binary cross entropy loss function, whereas the generator has been trained to minimize it. Because the generator has no idea about what kind of input it will receive from the discriminator, it must learn how to fool it by looking for a point on the latent space that maximizes its likelihood of producing this input. We can train GANs in this manner even without a ground-truth low-resolution image.

In our SR-GANN application, we attempted to perform image super resolution on X-ray images of patients. The architecture of the custom-designed SR-GANN for image super resolution is determined primarily by the generator design. The system's discriminator remains the same as in the proposed paper of the SR-GANN. The poly-amorous multi-perceptron layers are a special structure in the generator that comes before the residual connections. These are the primary feature-capture layers of the input images. The images are all X-ray images of patients, and the dataset contains approximately 5,000 images. Figure 7.4 presents the entire architecture of the generator of the SR-GANN for X-ray image super resolution.

The image super resolution generator is made up of custom-designed bi-modal multi-perceptron layers for capturing the features of low-resolution images; in our case, we used 5,000 images, each with a dimension of 16×16. The capture of features is critical during the super resolution of X-ray images. We used 50 residual blocks in the generator, each consisting of a convolutional layer, followed by batch normalization layers and PReLU layers, and finally the element-wise-summation layer. Residual blocks capture more details at a deeper level, and as proposed in the original Residual Networks paper, these techniques reduce the chances of over-fitting. In the generator of the SR-GANN, we did not use the Leaky Rectified Linear Unit Activation Function (LeakyReLU), rather we used the Parametric Rectified Linear Unit (PReLU), which ensures different slopes for predefined number of input features.

The discriminator network design of the SR-GANN system is shown in Figure 7.5. The discriminator is still in the same form as it was in the original publication. The discriminator in any type of GANN is used to assess whether or not the generated image from the generator is approaching the real images. The discriminator can be thought of as a binary classifier that can distinguish between authentic photos and artificially created fraudulent images. Deep CNNs with leaky rectified linear units as the internal activation function make up our specially created discriminator.

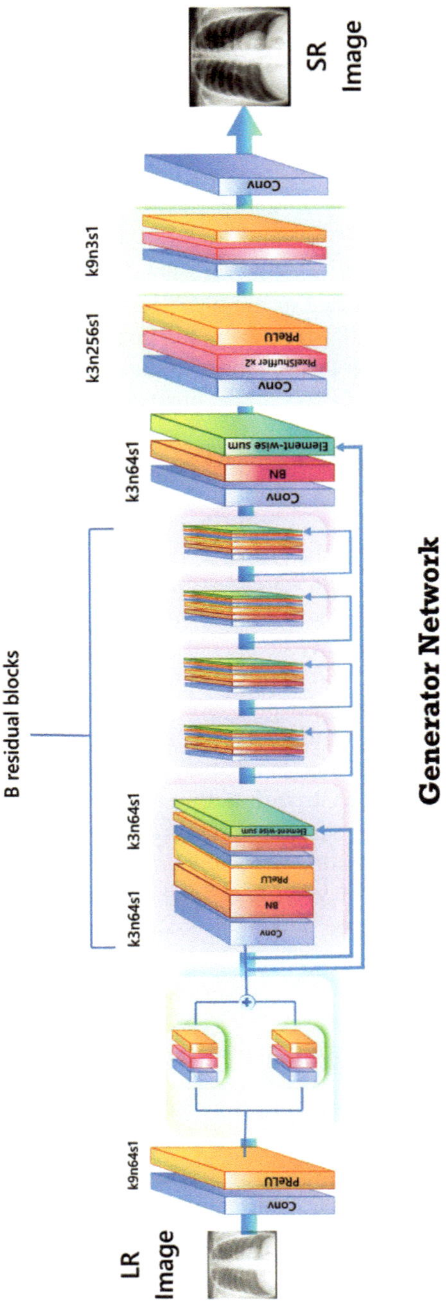

FIGURE 7.3 The generator of the X-ray image super resolution generative adversarial neural network with the bi-modal multi-perceptron layers incorporated at the beginning of the network.

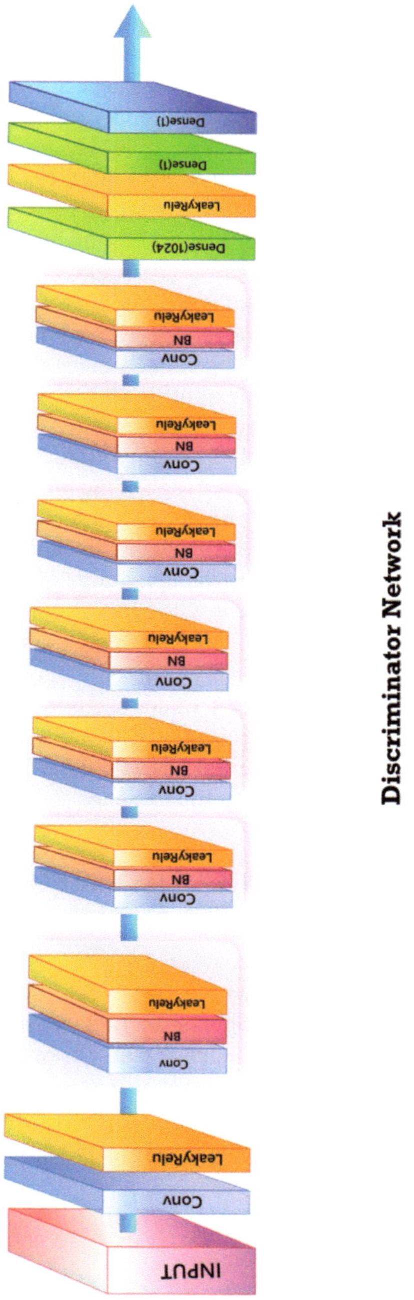

FIGURE 7.4 The Architecture of the discriminator of the X-ray image super resolution generative adversarial neural network.

A tensor with the dimensions [5000 ×16 × 16 × 1] is the generator's input, with 16×16×1 standing in for each low-resolution image and 5,000 representing the total number of photos. When using Super Resolution, the low-resolution photos are upscaled to values that are roughly square with the low-resolution values, or 256×256×1. The generator-generated higher resolution images with a dimension of 256×256×1 and the corresponding real high-resolution images are the input to the discriminator. A series of convolutional layers, fully connected layers, pooling layers, and ReLU non-linear layers are used to construct both the generator and the discriminator.

The generator is trained using targets that are batch size 256×256×1 images from ground-truth high-resolution photographs, which were randomly cropped from low-resolution images and randomly scaled between 0.5 and 2 times the original size. Ninety percent of the randomly cropped low-resolution photos are utilized for training and 10 percent are used for validation throughout each training iteration, which lasts for 30 epochs. At each training iteration, the generator generates images with a batch size of 256×256×1, and the discriminator is trained using a random cropping of both real high-resolution images and ground-truth high-resolution images, with a ratio of 5:1 (i.e., 5 samples from generator/1 sample from ground truth). Of the samples, 75% are used for training and 25% for validation for each of the 30 training iterations. Both discriminator CNNs are trained using boosting, with an increase in iterations (from 100 to 200) per 50 epochs. This is done because when discriminators trained on short datasets are fed into a GAN generator, the results on large datasets are inconsistent. The initial mixture weights had a zero mean Gaussian distribution, and throughout training, noise was added to change them. For example, to generate a new image at any scale, we can pick up 256 pixels randomly from one image as our starting point and then add noise by multiplying it by 0 or 1 values according to probability parameter p=0.5 or p=0.5+noise, respectively, such that most of the time we end up adding noise instead of multiplying by zero value (which will result in no change). We can then crop these lower resolution images into square shape.

7.4 IMPLEMENTATION OF THE X-RAY IMAGE SUPER RESOLUTION GENERATIVE NEURAL NETWORK SYSTEM

We will look at the SR-GANN implementation from scratch in Python by using Tensorflow. First, we will prepare the dataset for the low resolution as well as the higher resolution. The low-resolution image tensor is of the shape [5000 × 16 × 16 × 1] and the corresponding high-resolution image tensor is of the shape [5000 × 256 × 256 × 1]. For preparing the dataset, we created a function for the same in Python that uses some of the wonderful libraries, such as OpenCV, Numpy, OS, and others. The data preprocessing and preparation function implementation is provided below.

Source Code:

```
"import cv2"
"import numpy as np"
"import os"
"import matplotlib.pyplot as plt"
"from tqdm import tqdm"
```

```
"def generateDatasetForSRGann(train_dir,low_res_dir,high_
res_dir,low_res_size, high_res_size):"
    "for img in tqdm(os.listdir(train_dir)):"
        "img_array = cv2.imread(train_dir+"/"+img)"
        "high_res_img_array = cv2.resize(img_array, high_
res_size, cv2.INTER_LINEAR)"
        "low_res_img_array = cv2.resize(img_array,low_res_
size, cv2.INTER_LINEAR)"
        "cv2.imwrite(low_res_dir+"/"+img, low_res_img_array)"
        "cv2.imwrite(high_res_dir+"/"+img, high_res_img_array)"

"train_directory = ""  "
"save_low_path = ""  "
"save_high_path = ""  "

"generateDatasetForSRGann(train_directory, save_low_path,
save_high_path, (16, 16), (256, 256))"
```

The parameters for the data preparation function include the path to the training directory containing all the images, the path where both the low-resolution and high-resolution images will be saved, as well as the desired dimensions for the low-resolution (16×16) and high-resolution (256×256) images. This function utilizes OpenCV and NumPy to create the images one by one.

With the data preparation step completed, we can now proceed to design the SR-GAN using TensorFlow and Keras. It is essential to note that altering the image dimensions may require a substantial amount of RAM and GPU memory. We conducted this implementation on a system equipped with 128 GB of RAM and an Nvidia Tesla V-100 GPU with 24 GB of GPU memory. Running this code on a low-end system may result in performance issues or excessive power consumption.

We will now implement the SR-GAN architecture from scratch, including both the generator and the discriminator. We have designed two functions that internally utilize other custom-defined functions to create the structure of these components. Our implementation relies on TensorFlow and Keras to create an AI system capable of generating higher-resolution images from their lower-resolution counterparts.

Source Code:

```
"import os"
"import cv2"
"import numpy as np"
"from matplotlib import pyplot as plt"
"import tensorflow.keras as keras"
"from keras.models import Sequential"
"from keras import layers, Model"
"from keras.layers import Conv2D, PReLU, LeakyReLU,
BatchNormalization, Flatten"
"from keras.layers import UpSampling2D, Dense, Input, add"
"from tqdm import tqdm"
"from tensorflow.keras.optimizers import Adam, Nadam"
```

```
"from tensorflow.keras.applications import InceptionV3,
VGG19, VGG16"

"train_directory = ""  "
"save_low_path = ""  "
"save_high_path = ""  "

# The Residual Block of the SR-Gann
"def residualBlock(i_p, interpolate_layers):"
    "res_model = Conv2D(64, (3,3), padding='same', use_bias=
True, kernel_initializer='he_normal')(i_p)"
    "res_model = BatchNormalization(momentum=0.65)(res_model)"
    "res_model = PReLU(shared_axes = [1, 2])(res_model)"
    "if interpolate_layers == True:"
        "res_model = Conv2D(64, (3,3), padding='same', use_
bias=True, kernel_initializer='he_normal')(res_model)"
        "res_model = BatchNormalization(momentum=0.65)(res_
model)"
        "res_model = PReLU(shared_axes = [1, 2])(res_model)"
        "elif interpolate_layers == False:"
        "res_model = Conv2D(64, (3,3), padding='same', use_
bias=True, kernel_initializer='he_normal')(res_model)"
        "res_model = BatchNormalization(momentum=0.65)(res_
model)"
        "res_model = Conv2D(64, (3,3), padding='same')(res_
model)"
        "res_model = BatchNormalization(momentum=0.65)(res_
model)"

        "res_model_final = add([i_p, res_model])"

        "return res_model_final"

"def upscalingBlock(i_p):"
    "up_model = Conv2D(256, (3,3), padding='same')(i_p)"
    "up_model = UpSampling2D(size=(2,2), interpolation=
'nearest')(up_model)"
    "up_model = PReLU(shared_axes=[1, 2])(up_model)"
    "return up_model"

# Let us create the DCNN Residual Generator of the Super-
Resolution GANN
"def generatorSRGannFunction(input_generator, num_residual_
block):"
    "layers = Conv2D(64, (9,9), padding='same', kernel_
initializer='he_normal')(input_generator)"
    "layers = PReLU(shared_axes=[1, 2])(layers)"

    "control = layers"

    "for i in range(num_residual_block):"
        "layers = residualBlock(layers, True)"
    "layers = Conv2D(64, (3,3), padding='same', kernel_
initializer='he_normal')(layers)"
    "layers = BatchNormalization(momentum=0.65)(layers)"
```

```
    "layers = add([layers, control])"

    "layers = upscalingBlock(layers)"
    "layers = upscalingBlock(layers)"
    "layers = upscalingBlock(layers)"
    "layers = upscalingBlock(layers)"

    "output = Conv2D(3, (9,9), padding='same', kernel_
initializer='he_normal')(layers)"

    "return Model(inputs=input_generator, outputs=output)"

# The custom Convolutional layer for the discriminator block
"def discriminatorConvBlock(i_p, filters, strides=1, use_bn=True):"
    "disc_model = Conv2D(filters, (3,3), strides=strides,
padding='same')(i_p)"
    "if use_bn:"
        "disc_model = BatchNormalization(momentum=0.85)(disc_model)"
    "disc_model = LeakyReLU(alpha=0.17)(disc_model)"
"return disc_model"

# The Discriminator NEtwork of the SR-GANN
"def discriminatorSRGannFunction(input_discriminator, num_
filter_loop=64):"
    "df = num_filter_loop"

    "d1 = discriminatorConvBlock(input_discriminator, df,
use_bn=False)"
    "d2 = discriminatorConvBlock(d1, df, strides=2)"
    "d3 = discriminatorConvBlock(d2, df*2)"
    "d4 = discriminatorConvBlock(d3, df*2, strides=2)"
    "d5 = discriminatorConvBlock(d4, df*4)"
    "d6 = discriminatorConvBlock(d5, df*4, strides=2)"
    "d7 = discriminatorConvBlock(d6, df*8)"
    "d8 = discriminatorConvBlock(d7, df*8, strides=2)"

    "d8_1_flatten_layer = Flatten()(d8)"

    "d9 = Dense(df*16, kernel_initializer='he_normal')(d8_1_
flatten_layer)"
    "d10 = LeakyReLU(alpha=0.17)(d9)"

    "validity = Dense(1, activation='sigmoid', use_bias=True)(d10)"

    "return Model(input_discriminator, validity)"
```

First, we have created a function that would incorporate the residual blocks having convolution, batch normalization, parametric ReLU activation, element wise summation. This residual function is being called when we will be creating the generator network architecture. The upscaling block is also a part of the generator of the SR-GANN and thus plays the penultimate upscaling of the pixels and ensures perfect image super resolution. We have created a function for creating the generator network named as the "generatorSRGannFunction" that would internally use the residual blocks and upscaling blocks for the creation of the generator network of the proposed system.

The discriminator network of the SR-GANN is also developed using a function named as the "discriminatorSRGannFunction" that internally uses the discriminator's convolutional block that is having Leaky ReLU as the activation function along with convolutional layers incorporated with batch normalization. The discriminator that we have designed is slightly different than the original paper, as the original paper used a smaller less deep discriminator, but ours is a bit deeper for better capturing details during the training of the system.

In SR-GANN, the original paper mentions the incorporation of a perceptual loss factor by using another state-of-the-art algorithm that is capable of understanding features due to its pretrained weights on ImageNet. The network that we have used is the VGG19 model. Figure 7.5 presents the architecture of the VGG Model; the smaller variant has a total of 16 layers while the later has a total of 19 layers. The layers of the VGG are convolution layers and max pooling layers.

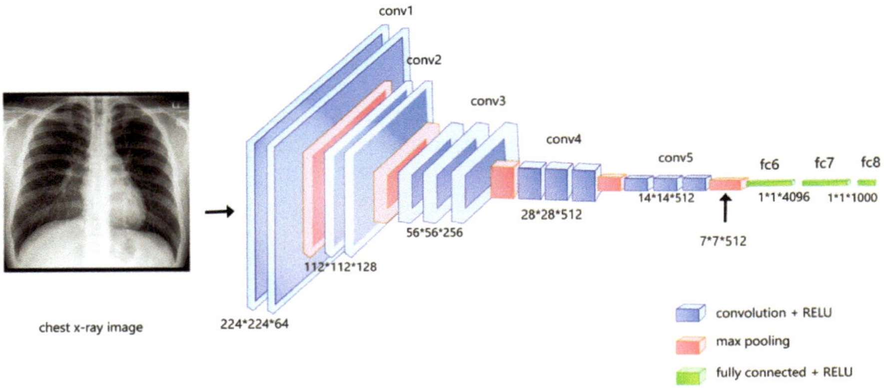

FIGURE 7.5 The VGG19 model for capturing the features present in the high-resolution images for acting as the perceptual loss component for better conversion of low-resolution images to higher resolution.

This VGG19 designed by us was the main source of calculating the perceptual loss during the training of the entire AI system. The generator of the SR-GANN basically tries to generate new higher resolution images from its corresponding low-resolution ones and thus during this training, the VGG19 also gets the generator's generated high-resolution images for matching the features of the real high-resolution images and the generator's ones. Thus, the VGG19 basically guides the generator of the SR-GANN toward minimizing the corresponding losses of perception via feature matching. The VGG19 can be treated as a feature extractor that would be working upon the generator's generated high-resolution images and the real high-resolution images. We have again created a function that would help us to access the VGG19 via Transfer Learning with Tensorflow. So, let us have a look at the implemented function. In the entire SR-GANN system, basically we are going to pass three inputs, the first one being the generator, the second one is the discriminator, and finally the VGG19 model that we have accessed using the aforementioned function.

Thus, we can have a look at how we have created the entire SR-GANN system, comprising the generator, discriminator, and VGG19 altogether.

Source Code:

```
"def VGG19ModelFunction(high_res_shape):"
    "vgg19 = VGG19(weights='imagenet', include_top=False,
input_shape=high_res_shape)"

    "return Model(inputs=vgg19.inputs, outputs=vgg19.
layers[10].output)"

# The Combined Model with VGG16
"def combinedModelWithVGG19Function(generator_model,
discriminator_model, vgg_model, low_res_input, high_res_input):"
    "gen_image = generator_model(low_res_input)"
    "gen_features = vgg_model(gen_image)"

    "discriminator_model.trainable = False"
    "validity = discriminator_model(gen_image)"

    "return Model(inputs=[low_res_input, high_res_input],
outputs=[validity, gen_features])"
```

The "VGG19ModelFunction" is the custom-designed function that we have created to access pretrained VGG19 model, via Tensorflow. The function requires a positional argument, "high_res_shape." The value that is being passed to this parameter was (256×256), as we are going to perform super resolution of images from 16×16 to 256×256. The "combinedModelWithVGG19Function" is the function that basically creates the entire super resolution GANN system with the positional arguments as the designed generator model, discriminator model, vgg19 model, low-resolution shape, and the high-resolution shape. In the VGG19 we use the layers till the tenth index but now till the last one. This parameter can be changed and experimented accordingly. For this experiment it is advised to keep the value less than 15 for better generation of super resolution images.

Now we are going to see how we have created the data processing, converting the images to the corresponding Numpy arrays for training the SR-GANN. We are using the dataset that we have used in the previous chapters for performing classification and detection. The images were first converted to the training low-resolution shapes and corresponding high-resolution shapes. Using OpenCV in Python we can easily perform image preprocessing and resizing as well. Let's have a look at the Python code for performing the image data preprocessing.

Source Code:

```
"train_directory = "Chest-Xray-SR-GANN-Dataset"  "
"save_low_path = "low-res-16-16-images"  "
"save_high_path = "high-res-256-256-images"  "

"low_res_dir = save_low_path"
"high_res_dir = save_high_path"
"list_low_res = os.listdir(low_res_dir)"
"list_high_res = os.listdir(high_res_dir)"

"print("Performing conversion for low-res images..")"
"lr_images = []"
```

```
"for image in tqdm(list_low_res):"
    "img_lr = cv2.imread(low_res_dir+"/"+image)"
    "lmg_lr = cv2.cvtColor(img_lr, cv2.COLOR_BGR2RGB)"
    "lr_images.append(img_lr)"

"print("Performing conversion for high-res images..")"
"hr_images = []"
"for image in tqdm(list_high_res):"
    "img_hr = cv2.imread(high_res_dir+"/"+image)"
    "img_hr = cv2.cvtColor(img_hr, cv2.COLOR_BGR2RGB)"
    "hr_images.append(img_hr)"

"low_res_images_array = np.array(lr_images)"
"high_res_images_array = np.array(hr_images)"

print(f"The shape of low resolution data array is :{low_res_
images_array.shape}")
print(f"The shape of high resolution data array is :{high_
res_images_array.shape}")
```

Console Output:

```
Performing conversion for low-res images..
100%|██████████| 5216/5216 [01:18<00:00, 66.13it/s]
Performing conversion for high-res images..
100%|██████████| 5216/5216 [25:47<00:00,  3.37it/s]
The shape of low-resolution data array is : (5216, 16, 16, 3)
The shape of high-resolution data array is : (5216, 256, 256, 3)
```

FIGURE 7.6 The output of the Python code. The shapes of the low-resolution and high-resolution tensors are provided that we will be using for the training of the SR-GANN.

Once we have converted the entire dataset into the corresponding low-resolution and high-resolution Numpy arrays or tensors, we can now plot some of the images together for a sanity checking so as to ensure proper image preprocessing. We will use the matplotlib library of Python for performing the plots of the data. Let's have a look at the dataset that we will be working with in the later stages.

Source Code:

```
"import random"
"import numpy as np"
"image_number = random.randint(0, len(lr_images)-1)"
"plt.figure(figsize=(12,6))"
"plt.subplot(121)"
"plt.imshow(np.reshape(low_res_images_array[image_number],
(16, 16, 3)))"
"plt.subplot(122)"
"plt.imshow(np.reshape(high_res_images_array[image_number],
(256, 256, 3)))"
"plt.show()"
```

Console Output:

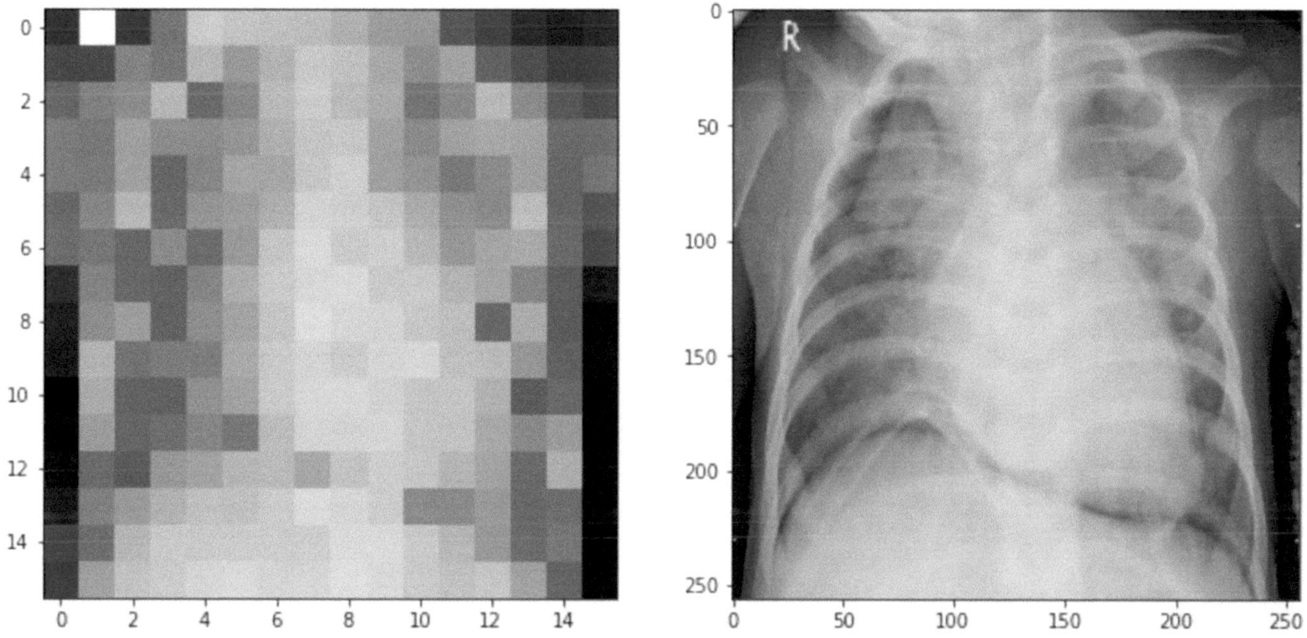

FIGURE 7.7 The low-resolution image of an X-ray with its corresponding high-resolution image.

Thus, as we have mentioned earlier, the images that we are going to work with are the images combined from previous chapters of this book. The low-resolution images have a custom dimension of 16×16 and the corresponding high-resolution images have a dimension of 256×256, as depicted in Figure 7.7. Now we will look at the utilization of the custom-defined functions for generating the entire system of SR-GANN. In creating the system of SR-GANN we will be using the functions that we have created for generating the generator, the discriminator, and many other required conditions. The advantage of creating custom functions for the generation of neural networks can be utilized to a great extent in Python as creating functions in Python can lead to easier and robust applications. Furthermore, we have provided implementation details of the corresponding function that we are going to apply in the coming sections. It is recommended that the default values must not be tampered during individual execution of the code. We have also provided the code for dividing the entire tensor that we have obtained for the low-resolution images and high-resolution images to the training and validation data tensor. Using the sklearn library of Python we will create the code for splitting the dataset Numpy array.

Source Code:

```
"low_res_images_array = low_res_images_array / 255.0"
"high_res_images_array = high_res_images_array / 255.0"

"from sklearn.model_selection import train_test_split"
"lr_train, lr_test, hr_train, hr_test = train_test_
split(low_res_images_array,
      high_res_images_array,
      test_size=0.25,
      random_state=42)"

"low_res_shape = (lr_train.shape[1], lr_train.shape[2], lr_
train.shape[3])"
"high_res_shape = (hr_train.shape[1], hr_train.shape[2], hr_
train.shape[3])"
"print("The low resolution shape and high resolution shape are :
{} and {} respectively".format(low_res_shape, high_res_shape))"
```

As we have completed the splitting of the training and validation Numpy data arrays, now we can move on to the creation of the components of the X-ray image super resolution GANN in Python by utilizing the custom-designed functions for creating the generator, discriminator, and VGG19 combined system. First, we will be creating the generator, with the help of the function that we have designed previously, the "generatorSRGannFunction." Here in this section we will be experimenting the robustness of Python functions for solving problems as well.

Source Code:

```
"from tensorflow.keras.utils import plot_model"
"lr_ip = Input(shape=low_res_shape)"
```

```
"hr_ip = Input(shape=high_res_shape)"
"generator = generatorSRGannFunction(lr_ip, num_residual_
block=50)"
"discriminator = discriminatorSRGannFunction(hr_ip)"
"discriminator.compile(loss='binary_crossentropy',
optimizer=Adam(learning_rate=0.001), metrics=['accuracy'])"
```

Thus, the Discriminator and the Generator networks are created and stored in the variables named as "generator" and "discriminator". Now we will be incorporating the perceptual loss via applying the VGG19 model that we will be accessing using the predefined functions.

Source Code:

```
"vgg19 = VGG19ModelFunction((256, 256, 3))"
"vgg19.summary()"
"vgg19.trainable = False"
```

Console Output: -

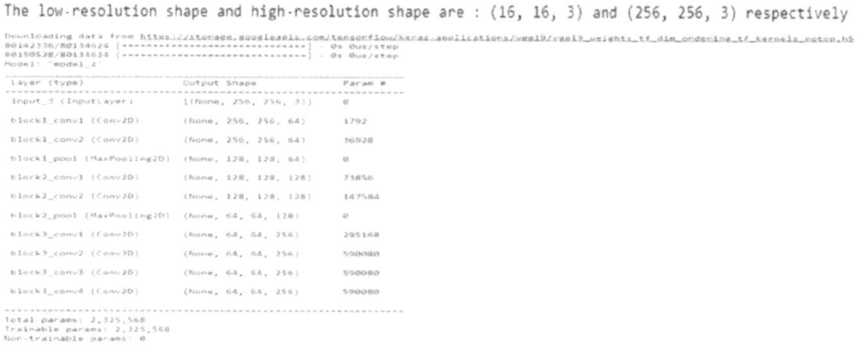

```
The low-resolution shape and high-resolution shape are : (16, 16, 3) and (256, 256, 3) respectively

Downloading data from https://storage.googleapis.com/tensorflow/keras-applications/vgg19/vgg19_weights_tf_dim_ordering_tf_kernels_notop.h5
80142336/80134624 [==============================] - 0s 0us/step
80150528/80134624 [==============================] - 0s 0us/step
Model: "model_2"
_________________________________________________________________
 Layer (type)                Output Shape              Param #
=================================================================
 input_3 (InputLayer)        [(None, 256, 256, 3)]     0

 block1_conv1 (Conv2D)       (None, 256, 256, 64)      1792

 block1_conv2 (Conv2D)       (None, 256, 256, 64)      36928

 block1_pool (MaxPooling2D)  (None, 128, 128, 64)      0

 block2_conv1 (Conv2D)       (None, 128, 128, 128)     73856

 block2_conv2 (Conv2D)       (None, 128, 128, 128)     147584

 block2_pool (MaxPooling2D)  (None, 64, 64, 128)       0

 block3_conv1 (Conv2D)       (None, 64, 64, 256)       295168

 block3_conv2 (Conv2D)       (None, 64, 64, 256)       590080

 block3_conv3 (Conv2D)       (None, 64, 64, 256)       590080

 block3_conv4 (Conv2D)       (None, 64, 64, 256)       590080

=================================================================
Total params: 2,325,568
Trainable params: 2,325,568
Non-trainable params: 0
```

FIGURE 7.8 The VGG19 model that we will be using for the perceptual loss calculation but we have used layers till the tenth index.

Thus, we have again used the predefined functions for the creation of the required perceptual loss calculation via, the VGG19 model as depicted in Figure 7.8. We have used the VGG19 model till the 10th layer and, hence, the model was capable of providing enough details that can be treated as a mean for storing the perceptual loss. Now we will be incorporating this VGG19 model stored in the variable named as vgg19 in the system of the SR-GANN again by utilizing the combined model function. The VGG19 part that we are using consists of around 2 million (M) parameters and when on creation of the SR-GANN system, these parameters would be added as total parameters. In the generator, the total parameters were around 7 M and the discriminator was having a total parameter of around 138 M.

Source Code:

```
"gan_model = combinedModelWithVGG19Function(generator,
                                             discriminator,
                                             vgg19, lr_ip, hr_
                                             ip)"

"gan_model.compile(loss=['binary_crossentropy', 'mse'],
                   loss_weights=[1e-3, 1],
                   optimizer=Adam(learning_rate=
                   0.0003))"

"gan_model.summary()"
```

Console Output:

```
Model: "model_3"
__________________________________________________________________________________________________
 Layer (type)                   Output Shape         Param #     Connected to
==================================================================================================
 input_1 (InputLayer)           [(None, 16, 16, 3)]  0           []

 model (Functional)             (None, 256, 256, 3)  3709251     ['input_1[0][0]']

 input_2 (InputLayer)           [(None, 256, 256, 3  0           []
                                )]

 model_1 (Functional)           (None, 1)            138912577   ['model[0][0]']

 model_2 (Functional)           (None, 64, 64, 256)  2325568     ['model[0][0]']

==================================================================================================
Total params: 144,947,396
Trainable params: 3,703,363
Non-trainable params: 141,244,033
__________________________________________________________________________________________________
```

FIGURE 7.9 The entire SR-GANN system comprising the generator, the discriminator, and the perceptual loss calculator, the VGG19 model altogether.

The entire system that we have designed for the super resolution of X-ray images now is stored in a variable named as the "gan_model." The generator, the discriminator, and the vgg19 are components of the SR-GANN. The non-trainable parameters that were present in the entire combined system are due to the presence of numerous batch normalization layers that contribute to the same. Thus, we have created our application-specific SR-GANN for the application on X-ray images as depicted in Figure 7.9 in details. The combined model would be trained now upon the dataset arrays and, thus, we will be able to generate new higher resolution images from low-resolution ones. The system is capable of performing super resolution at a very large scale and also to a higher resolution value. In our experiment we have tried to perform super resolution on images having dimensions of 16×16 and generated images of higher resolution size of 256×256. The training of the GANN was totally same as that of any traditional GANN and hence we will be implementing it from scratch in Python using TensorFlow and Keras. The entire network was trained for around 5,000 epochs using a batch size of 1. The system that was used for the training of the network consists of a RAM of 128 GB and a Tesla V100 GPU. Figure 7.10 depicts the ongoing training of the designed SR-GANN system. Normal systems are not recommended for the execution of the training. Using Google Collab Pro+ can be a solution but the performance can differ. While the network is getting trained, we have saved certain checkpointed models for performing inferences later on.

Source Code:

```
"batch_size = 1"
"epochs = 5000"

"train_lr_batches = []"
"train_hr_batches = []"
"for item in tqdm(range(int(hr_train.shape[0] / batch_
size))):"
    "start_idx = item * batch_size"
    "end_idx = start_idx + batch_size"
    "train_hr_batches.append(hr_train[start_idx:end_idx])"
    "train_lr_batches.append(lr_train[start_idx:end_idx])"

# Enumerate Training over epochs
"for e in range(epochs):"
    "fake_label = np.zeros((batch_size, 1))"
    "real_label = np.ones((batch_size, 1))"

    # Lists for storing the losses matrix for inferences
    "generator_loss = []"
    "discriminator_loss = []"

    # Enumerate training over batches
    "for b in tqdm(range(len(train_hr_batches))):"
         "lr_imgs = train_lr_batches[b]"
         "hr_imgs = train_hr_batches[b]"

         # Generator Generating Fake images
         "fake_imgs = generator.predict_on_batch(lr_imgs)"

         # Training the discriminator first on real and fake HR Images
         "discriminator.trainable = True"
         "discriminator_loss_gen   =   discriminator.train_on_
batch(fake_imgs, fake_label)"
         "discriminator_loss_real   =   discriminator.train_on_
batch(hr_imgs, real_label)"

         # Training the generator by fixing the discriminator
as non-trainable
         "discriminator.trainable = False"

         # Averageing the discriminator losses
         "d_loss = 0.5 * np.add(discriminator_loss_gen, dis-
criminator_loss_real)"
```

```
        # Extracting VGG16 Features for the perceptual loss application
        "image_features = vgg19.predict(hr_imgs)"

        # Train the generator via the GANN Model
        # With 2 losses,
        # 1) the adverserial loss (Binary-Crossentropy)
        # 2) the content loss (VGG Loss, MSE)

        "g_loss, _, _ = gan_model.train_on_batch([lr_imgs,
hr_imgs], [real_label, image_features])"
        "generator_loss.append(g_loss)"
        "discriminator_loss.append(d_loss)"

        # Converting the lists to the corresponding numpy
arrays for adding
        "generator_loss = np.array(generator_loss)"
        "discriminator_loss = np.array(discriminator_loss)"

        # Calculating the average losses for the generator
and discriminator
        "g_loss = np.sum(generator_loss, axis=0) / len(generator_
loss)"
        "d_loss = np.sum(discriminator_loss, axis=0) / len(discriminator_
loss)"

        # Reporting the progress while training
        "print(f"Epoch : {e + 1}, with Generator Loss : {g_
loss}, and Discriminator Losses : {d_loss[0]} on fake and {d_
loss[1]} on real")"

        "if (e + 1) % 5 == 0:"
            "generator.save("Xray-SR-GANN-Models-2/gen_e_"
+ str(e + 1) + ".h5")"
```

Console Output:

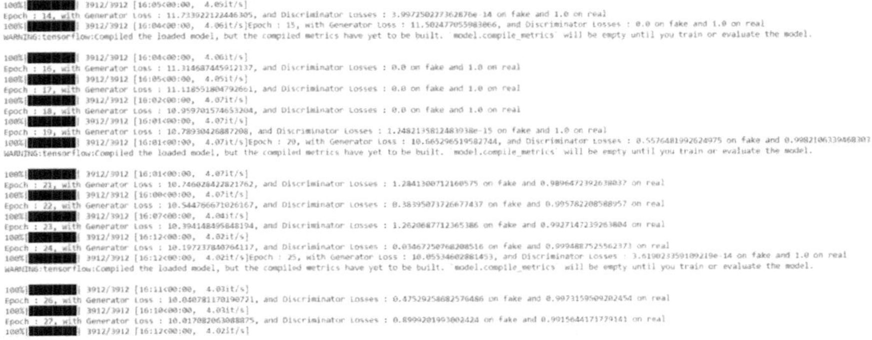

```
100%|██████████| 3912/3912 [16:02<00:00,  4.06it/s]
Epoch : 11, with Generator Loss : 12.64074561993281, and Discriminator Losses : 1.4377443848577898 on fake and 0.9888803680981595 on real
100%|██████████| 3912/3912 [16:04<00:00,  4.06it/s]
Epoch : 12, with Generator Loss : 12.258556016444672, and Discriminator Losses : 0.050737250070682464 on fake and 0.9993609406052960 on real
100%|██████████| 3912/3912 [16:04<00:00,  4.06it/s]
Epoch : 13, with Generator Loss : 11.972586319246663, and Discriminator Losses : 1.7954777159961346e-34 on fake and 1.0 on real
100%|██████████| 3912/3912 [16:05<00:00,  4.05it/s]
Epoch : 14, with Generator Loss : 11.733922122446305, and Discriminator Losses : 3.997250227362876e-14 on fake and 1.0 on real
100%|██████████| 3912/3912 [16:04<00:00,  4.06it/s]Epoch : 15, with Generator Loss : 11.502477055983066, and Discriminator Losses : 0.0 on fake and 1.0 on real
WARNING:tensorflow:Compiled the loaded model, but the compiled metrics have yet to be built. `model.compile_metrics` will be empty until you train or evaluate the model.

100%|██████████| 3912/3912 [16:04<00:00,  4.06it/s]
Epoch : 16, with Generator Loss : 11.314687445912137, and Discriminator Losses : 0.0 on fake and 1.0 on real
100%|██████████| 3912/3912 [16:05<00:00,  4.05it/s]
Epoch : 17, with Generator Loss : 11.118551804792661, and Discriminator Losses : 0.0 on fake and 1.0 on real
100%|██████████| 3912/3912 [16:02<00:00,  4.07it/s]
Epoch : 18, with Generator Loss : 10.959701574653204, and Discriminator Losses : 0.0 on fake and 1.0 on real
100%|██████████| 3912/3912 [16:01<00:00,  4.07it/s]
Epoch : 19, with Generator Loss : 10.78930426887208, and Discriminator Losses : 1.2482135812483938e-15 on fake and 1.0 on real
100%|██████████| 3912/3912 [16:01<00:00,  4.07it/s]Epoch : 20, with Generator Loss : 10.665296519582744, and Discriminator Losses : 0.5576481992624975 on fake and 0.9982106339468303
WARNING:tensorflow:Compiled the loaded model, but the compiled metrics have yet to be built. `model.compile_metrics` will be empty until you train or evaluate the model.

100%|██████████| 3912/3912 [16:01<00:00,  4.07it/s]
Epoch : 21, with Generator Loss : 10.746028422821762, and Discriminator Losses : 1.2841300712160575 on fake and 0.9896472392638037 on real
100%|██████████| 3912/3912 [16:00<00:00,  4.07it/s]
Epoch : 22, with Generator Loss : 10.544766671026167, and Discriminator Losses : 0.38395073726677437 on fake and 0.995782208588957 on real
100%|██████████| 3912/3912 [16:07<00:00,  4.04it/s]
Epoch : 23, with Generator Loss : 10.394148495848194, and Discriminator Losses : 1.2620687712365386 on fake and 0.9927147239263804 on real
100%|██████████| 3912/3912 [16:12<00:00,  4.02it/s]
Epoch : 24, with Generator Loss : 10.197237840764117, and Discriminator Losses : 0.03467250768208516 on fake and 0.9994887525562373 on real
100%|██████████| 3912/3912 [16:12<00:00,  4.02it/s]Epoch : 25, with Generator Loss : 10.05534602881453, and Discriminator Losses : 3.619023359109219e-14 on fake and 1.0 on real
WARNING:tensorflow:Compiled the loaded model, but the compiled metrics have yet to be built. `model.compile_metrics` will be empty until you train or evaluate the model.

100%|██████████| 3912/3912 [16:11<00:00,  4.03it/s]
Epoch : 26, with Generator Loss : 10.040781170190721, and Discriminator Losses : 0.47529258682576486 on fake and 0.9973159509202454 on real
100%|██████████| 3912/3912 [16:10<00:00,  4.03it/s]
Epoch : 27, with Generator Loss : 10.017082063088875, and Discriminator Losses : 0.8999201993002424 on fake and 0.9915644171779141 on real
100%|██████████| 3912/3912 [16:12<00:00,  4.02it/s]
```

FIGURE 7.10 The training of the designed SR-GANN.

Now we will be performing the inferences on the testing dataset by the saved models that we have checkpointed during the training. For performing inferences, we have again used Tensorflow and Python along with Matplotlib to see the generated images and compare the loss or precision of generator as depicted in Figure 7.11. Thus, we have provided the code that would help us to perform the prediction and generation of images from low-resolution inputs.

Source Code:

```
"from keras.models import load_model"
"from numpy.random import randint"

"def plotPredictionsSRGann(model_path_sr_gann, figure_size):"
    "import warnings"
    "warnings.filterwarnings('ignore')"

    "model_path = model_path_sr_gann"
    "generator = load_model(filepath=model_path, compile=False)"

    "[X1, X2] = [lr_test, hr_test]"
    "ix = randint(0, len(X1), 1)"
    "src_image, target_image = X1[ix], X2[ix]"

    # Let the saved generator make the high-res prediction
    "generated_image = generator.predict(src_image)"
    # Let us see how the images look by plotting graphs
    "plt.figure(figsize=figure_size)"
    "plt.subplot(231)"
    "plt.title("Low-Resolution COVID X-ray Image")"
    "plt.imshow(src_image[0, :, :, :])"
    "plt.subplot(232)"
    "plt.title("Super-Resolution X-ray Image (SR-GANN)")"
    "plt.imshow(generated_image[0, :, :, :])"
    "plt.subplot(233)"
    "plt.title("Original High Resolution X-ray Image")"
    "plt.imshow(target_image[0, :, :, :])"

    "plt.show()"

" MODEL1 = "Xray-SR-GANN-Models-2/gen_e_5.h5" "
" MODEL2 = "Xray-SR-GANN-Models-2/gen_e_30.h5" "
" MODEL3 = "Xray-SR-GANN-Models-2/gen_e_50.h5" "

"plotPredictionsSRGann(MODEL2, (20,10))"
"plotPredictionsSRGann(MODEL2, (20,10))"
"plotPredictionsSRGann(MODEL2, (20,10))"
```

Console Output:

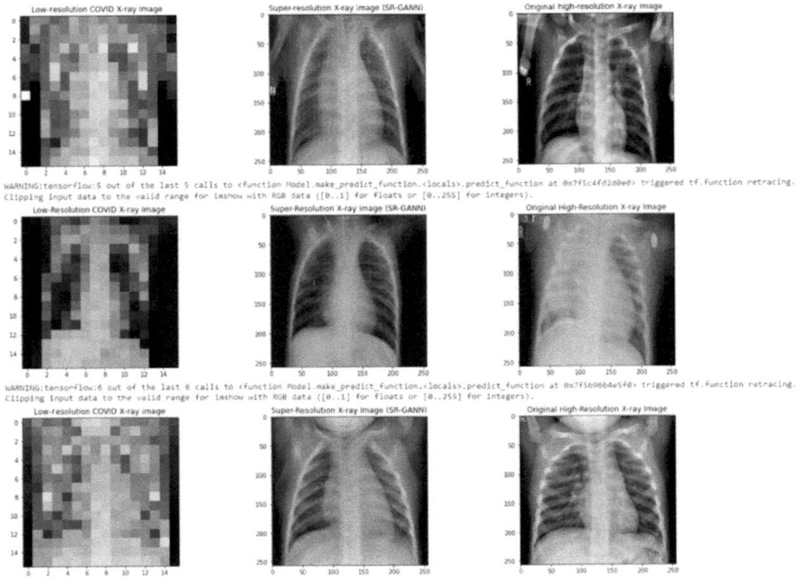

FIGURE 7.11 The generated super resolution X-ray images from low-resolution shape of 16×16 to a high-resolution shape of 256×256.

7.5 CONCLUSION

Thus, on having a closer look at the predictions by the models, we can say that the results were quite realistic. The generator was able to generate the super resolution images from their corresponding low-resolution ones and hence was able to up-sample the images to a great extent. The designed generator was able to perform the super resolution of the low-resolution images properly due to the presence of the bi-modal multi-perceptron layers at the beginning. The residual blocks were also responsible for the better generation of the feature maps as the VGG19 perceptual was incorporated. Our designed model system was able to perform super resolution of low-resolution images with quite ease as well as within few seconds. Nowadays, in hospitals the amount of data is getting increased exponentially. An image of an X-ray can have a size of around 10 MB but if we can store the images as the low-resolution version and then perform the super resolution with the desired SR-GANNs, then it would allow the hospitals to store a lot of images at a size of 16×16×1. Doctors or medical researchers can use our SR-GANN for performing super resolution upon the images and hence they can have an analysis of the images as well. Thus, using this principle of performing super resolution can be of a great help in the present hospitals. In future, we plan to use the SR-GANNs to perform super resolution of low-resolution medical images so that they can be utilized properly in the hospitals.

As we know, the size of the X-ray images is quite large, so if we can make use of the SR-GANNs to perform super resolution upon these images to get the high-resolution images, then it would be of a great help to the doctors to perform diagnostics at a much better level. Also, in the future, we plan to design the models by varying the number of perceptrons and the number of residual blocks and see the results to get the best model configuration. Moreover, we will also try to implement our proposed SR-GANNs on larger datasets as well as on other types of images to verify whether our proposed model is capable of doing super resolution for different types of images. In this experiment, we have proposed an advanced super resolution generative adversarial network called bi-modal multi-perceptron residual GANs (SR-GANNs) which is capable of performing super resolution of low-resolution images within few seconds. We have conducted various experiments to prove the validity of our proposed model system. We have implemented our proposed model system on various types of images such as animals and buildings. We have designed a generator with the help of the multiple perceptron layers which worked as the initializing layer for the other layers. We have applied the bi-modal multi-perceptron layers for the generation of the feature maps from the low-resolution images. We have used the concept of the residual blocks for the better generation of the feature maps as well as for the proper training of the model system. Moreover, we have used a VGG19 perceptual loss function for the better training of our model system. Our proposed model system was able to achieve the best results for the up-sampling of the low-resolution images. We have also implemented this model system on the large-sized images such as animals and buildings and were able to obtain the best results. In future, we plan to use the SR-GANNs to perform super resolution of low-resolution medical images so that they can be utilized properly in hospitals. As we know, the size of the X-ray images is quite large, so if we can make use of the SR-GANNs to perform super resolution upon these images to get the high-resolution images, then it would be of a great help to the doctors to perform diagnostics at a much better level. Also, in the future, we plan to design the models by varying the number of perceptrons and the number of residual blocks and see the results to get the best model configuration. Moreover, we will also try to implement our proposed SR-GANNs on larger datasets as well as on other types of images to verify whether our proposed model is capable of doing super resolution for different types of images.

REFERENCES

1. Goodfellow, I., Pouget-Abadie, J., Mirza, M., Xu, B., Warde-Farley, D., Ozair, S., Courville, A. and Bengio, Y., 2014. Generative adversarial nets. *Advances in Neural Information Processing Systems.*
2 Ledig, C., Theis, L., Huszár, F., Caballero, J., Cunningham, A., Acosta, A., Aitken, A., Tejani, A., Totz, J., Wang, Z. and Shi, W., 2017. Photo-realistic single image super-resolution using a generative adversarial network. In *Proceedings of the IEEE conference on computer vision and pattern recognition.*
3. Yang, W., Zhang, X., Tian, Y., Wang, W., Xue, J.H. and Liao, Q., 2019. Deep learning for single image super-resolution: A brief review. *IEEE Transactions on Multimedia*, 21(12), pp. 3106–3121.

4. Lim, B., Son, S., Kim, H., Nah, S. and Mu Lee, K., 2017. Enhanced deep residual networks for single image super-resolution. In *Proceedings of the IEEE conference on computer vision and pattern recognition workshops*.
5. Xu, L., Zeng, X., Huang, Z., Li, W. and Zhang, H., 2020. Low-dose chest X-ray image super-resolution using generative adversarial nets with spectral normalization. *Biomedical Signal Processing and Control*, 55, p. 101600.
6. Yu, Y., She, K. and Liu, J., 2021. Wavelet frequency separation attention network for chest X-ray image super-resolution. *Micromachines*, 12(11), p. 1418.
7. Amaranageswarao, G., Deivalakshmi, S. and Ko, S.B., 2020. Wavelet based medical image super resolution using cross connected residual-in-dense grouped convolutional neural network. *Journal of Visual Communication and Image Representation*, 70, p. 102819.
8. Radford, A., Metz, L. and Chintala, S., 2015. Unsupervised representation learning with deep convolutional generative adversarial networks. *arXiv preprint* arXiv:1511.06434.
9. Zhang, H., Goodfellow, I., Metaxas, D. and Odena, A., 2019, May. Self-attention generative adversarial networks. In *International conference on machine learning* (pp. 7354–7363).
10. Metz, L., Poole, B., Pfau, D. and Sohl-Dickstein, J., 2016. Unrolled generative adversarial networks. *arXiv preprint* arXiv:1611.02163.

8 Conclusion

The main concept of this book centers on the creation of medical application software that is able to carry out complex tasks. The book is written in such a way that reading it would be highly captivating for the reader. The first chapter focuses on the use of neural networks in science and research that is driven by medical data. The reader will be able to comprehend the ideas of deep learning, which is a subset of machine learning, starting in Chapter 2 and continuing through Chapter 4. Many additional complex algorithms, starting with convolutional neural networks (CNNs), were also included in the book, with a focus on solving various domain-specific applications. The readers of these chapters should be familiar with the fundamentals of Python programming and some of the basic ideas of deep learning. The chapters will also educate readers about the uses of neural networks in addition to guiding them toward a greater understanding of the subject. CNNs have essentially been used for a variety of tasks, including COVID-19 detection, chest X-ray classification, medical image reconstruction, and many others. Readers can also follow the chapters step by step to create the exact designed architectures. The use of the algorithms was also illustrated using the Python programming language. We have also developed illustrated visuals to illustrate key ideas, which call for specific advanced principles of conventional deep learning. These domain-specific neural networks were developed using Tensorflow, a well-known Python framework. The detailed implementation of lessons in these chapters also requires a familiarity with Tensorflow programming.

In Chapters 5, 6, and 7, which cover considerably more complex practical deep learning techniques, we attempted to develop interactive, adaptable models that could handle far more difficult jobs. The main focus of these chapters is to show how artificial neural networks can be applied to issues that are far more challenging than simple image classifications. In Chapter 7, we also used a specific kind of generative adversarial neural networks (GANNs). For the purpose of picture compression and subsequent image super resolution, we have developed an X-ray image super resolution GANN in this chapter. The 16×16 low-quality photos might be converted to 256×256 high-resolution images using the developed GANN. All readers would be able to comprehend how deep learning's complex algorithms can be used to advance medical data-driven science and research. Without being explicitly coded, deep learning algorithms are capable of automatically learning from experience

DOI: 10.1201/9781003456476-8

and enhancing themselves. This is a significant benefit over conventional machine learning techniques, which demand a lot of hand-curated data. Deep learning is also effective for unstructured or unlabeled data, including text, photos, and audio. Machine learning's field of deep learning is expanding quickly.

We hope that readers would be able to understand each topic covered in this book. Thus,

> AI and Computer Vision are the lenses through which we glimpse the future, a future where human potential knows no bounds. Together, they unlock the power to see what's invisible, understand the incomprehensible, and elevate human creativity and productivity to unprecedented heights. The fusion of technology and human ingenuity will redefine how we work, learn, and innovate, illuminating a path toward a brighter and more remarkable tomorrow.

Index

H

I

J

K

L

M